QUALITY IMPROVEMENT:

C3 IN ADVANCECARE PLANNING

A Gift of Clarity

Villeroy Akere Tah, DNP, RN.

Acknowledgments

The author acknowledges the contributions of the Elms College Faculty and DNP Capstone Project Experts and faculty advisors, especially Dr. Teresa Reske, Dr. Deborah Naglieri-Prescod, Dr. Lisa Wolf, and Dr. Majorie Childers for guiding the Elms Capstone Project Process Model through the successful implementation of this quality improvement project. The author acknowledges the support of Mr. Michael Fitzgerald, Clerk of Session of Hartford Street Presbyterian Church (HSPC) Natick MA, Reverend Katie Cote, the Pastor of HSPC, and the ruling body "Session of HSPC" for welcoming the project in their church and acting as liaisons with the congregants.

The author acknowledges the following health care professionals in the community; Maureen Kisob, BSN, RN, Cedonne Tah, MHS, and Jane Asembo, BSN, RN, for the support they provided during the implementation phase of the project. The author acknowledges peers at Elms College for the times they shared knowledge through classwork collaboration, and all those who shared their perspectives on the topic. The author acknowledges her Tah/Tamufor/Achu families, MbudcaNE family, Peers at Elms College, and the HSPC Community for their support during this time.

Dedication

This final Capstone Project idea through its implementation is dedicated to the author's husband (Mr. Richard Tah), children (Tamenang, Tifuh, Seta, and Kah) and mother (Esther Achu) who, daily, contributed to the author's physical, emotional, and intellectual well-being during my academic studies and this project. Lastly, to "Njango", who when caring for him gave me the inspiration to explore issues around advance care planning (ACP) among African American adults.

Contributors for the Quality Improvement Project (Part 1)

Dr. Teresa Kuta Reske—Elms College DNP Capstone Chair

Dr. Deborah Naglieri-Prescod, Elms College DNP Capstone Project Expert

Dr. Majorie Childers, Elms College DNP—Faculty Capstone Project Expert

Dr. Lisa Wolf, Elms College DNP Faculty

Mr. Michael Fitzgerald, Clerk of HSPC Natick

Reverend Katie Cote, Pastor of HSPC Natick

Ms. Maurine Kisob, BSN, RN, Community Nurse

Ms. Cedonne Tah, MSH, Behavioral Health Community Worker

Mrs. Jane Asembo, BSN, RN

Contributors for Testimonials:
African American Perspectives on Advance Directives (Part 2)
by first names only.

Sherlyn, Nurse (Liberian American)

Jane, Nurse (Kenyan American)

Evonne, PCA (Cameroonian American)

Lansana, Security Officer (Sierra Leonean American)

Louisa, Nurse (Ghanian American)

Vivian, Nurse (Ghanian American)

Calvin, Nurse (Cameroonian American)

Anonymous, Nurse (South African American)

Anonymous, Sales Associate (Moroccan American)

CONTENTS

PART 2: African American Perspectives on Advance Care Planning Discussions and Advance Directive Completion

PART 3: Systems Approach to Increasing Readiness to Engage in Advance Care Planning Discussions and Advance Directive Completion

PREFACE

The landscape of health care is constantly evolving with increased innovations in technological know-how. The once before wide world is not a global village. The ease of movement with people and the visual technology have enriched community experiences at different levels. Migrants traveled to other parts of the world before searching for "greener pasters" and often returned to their home countries. The increasing trend to have African immigrants in America has increased the pressure on complex health care needs like diabetes and hypertension management which have a high prevalence in the population. Personal conversations with a handful of African Americans who have been here for decades indicated that most thought their stay was temporal for work and school. They noted that America offers the things their home countries could not, employment, political instability, and transparency.

These immigrants (20–40 years ago) didn't focus on investing in real estate because they planned to return "home." Instead, they report they are just coming to realize that, regardless of the nostalgia often shared about their home country, America is their home now. This phenomenon is vital because HSB reported as "foreign" before maybe welcomed with increasing assimilation. For example, a typical response to Americans of descent is "it is not in our culture to plan for end-of-life care."

There is limited access to health care for African Americans from a systems view. However, if known to both the health professional and the population affected, the culture of care being rendered and expected respectively may arrive at a consensus for improved outcomes. However, structural issues are contributory factors to the continuous gap in health care. This book intends to explore modifiable factors within the African American population and utilize current resources in the community to reduce the gap while advocating for sound policies for public health sectors.

But more importantly, there is a disconnect when it comes to an understanding of the critical issues in the African American communities and the design of interventions tailored to these communities. Most studies do not target specific communities of color. "Black" is often used as an umbrella term for Americans with dark skin. There are, of course, cultural differences between Americans of African descent and other black Americans, which may skew data if not taken into consideration.

Part 1 of this book addresses status of ACP discussions and advance directive (AD) completion among African Americans from the health care professional's perspective. Evidence pointed to a gap in ACP and advance directive possession among "black" Americans. However, there was insufficient data or studies available to understand the extent among African Americans in particular.

Therefore, with the help of Elms College Faculty Staff, this author completed a quality improvement (QI) study in a faith-based community. The aim was to understand the congregants' status with ACP, initiate and increase ACP discussions, and increase AD possession among the participants.

Part 2 of this book is a collection of testimonials from Americans of African descent. They come from different works of life and voluntarily shared their viewpoint and experiences with Advance Directives (HCP, Wills, Power of Attorney). The author shares the first names of the interviewees with their permission.

Lastly, Part 3 of this book is a suggestive model of the Collaborative Cultural Competence (C3) in ACP, a framework to address the lower odds of ACP discussions and AD completion in the African American population. The model is also applicable for shared community and public health issues like vaccine hesitancy.

This book provides nursing scholars and advance practice nurses with the knowledge and skills needed to develop programs, projects, and health policies in this area, which may facilitate the realization of equitable health outcomes and just for all patients.

Furthermore, this book calls on nursing students and novice nurses to first understand their own cultural views on the ACP topic and seek cultural competence or skills training when addressing AD completion with their patients.

Lastly, this book provides an overview to African Americans about the issue at hand (low AD completion in their communities) and the importance of engaging in ACP conversations with family members and the health care profession.

Finally, for anyone looking for the best evidence-based practices to increase health care access to minority populations, I hope this book motivates you to incorporate the patient's perspective when planning for their care.

PART 1:

Quality Improvement Project

A Doctor of Nursing Practice Final Capstone Project

Submitted to the Doctor of Nursing Practice Faculty of the College of Our Lady of the Elms

In Partial Fulfillment for the Requirements of the Degree,

Doctor of Nursing Practice

By

Villeroy Tah MSN, RN

DNP Capstone Chairperson: Dr. Teresa Kuta Reske DNP, MPA, RN

DNP Capstone Team Member: Maurine Kisob BSN, RN

Spring 2022.

Improving Readiness in Advance Care Planning (ACP) Behaviors among African American Adults in the Community

Abstract

A quality improvement project was conducted with 30 African American adults with the goal of encouraging their familiarity with and completion of an Advance Directive (AD). Black Americans have been shown to have lower participation in Advanced Care Planning (ACP) than Whites or Hispanics. Records indicate that hospital patients without an AD have lower rates of invasive procedures, higher cost of care, and more extended hospital stays than those who have one. A multimodal (printed documents, live discussions, educational videos) intervention carried out in a Black faith-based setting presented information and discussion opportunities about choosing a Health Care Proxy (HCP) and how to discuss wishes and treatment preferences with family and healthcare providers, especially at end of life. Theoretical grounding came from Kolcaba's Comfort Theory combined with the Transtheoretical Model (TTM) by Prochaska and DiClemente. The Collaborative Cultural Competence (C3) framework was created to meet the needs of the QI project. Results of the project were that 23% (n =7) completed an HCP; 57% (17) indicated that they planned to complete one within three to six months. Overall, the project improved engagement in ACP behaviors by 47%, as reported by participants. The project also yielded information suggesting the complexity of this issue among African American adults and calls for additional research to better understand barriers to reducing the healthcare planning gap. Essential II from the American Association of Colleges of Nursing was demonstrated in this project by using systems thinking and healthcare organizations to encourage ACP behaviors in the African American population.

Keywords: advance care planning, advance care planning behaviors, advance directives, African Americans, multimodal presentations.

CHAPTER 1:

Improving Readiness in ACP Behaviors among African American Adults in the Community

Introduction

Advance directives are written statements by individuals on often standardized forms on which they express their wishes and preferences for treatment options should individuals become unable to make those decisions. Sixty-three percent (or 2 in 3) of American adults have not completed an AD (Yadav, Gabler, Cooney, Kent, Kim, Herst, Mante, Halpern, & Courtright, 2017). Huang, Neuheaus, and Chiong (2016) report White older adults (44.0 percent) are more likely to possess ADs than Hispanics (29%) and Black older adults (24%). Although there have been increased legislative and clinical efforts in the past decade to increase the completion of advance directives, extensive research findings continue to show a gap in ACP with Black American individuals.

Although this Doctor in Nursing Practice (DNP) student was unable to find ACP studies conducted exclusively among the African American population in the community setting, the findings from the vastly studied Black American population will help guide evidence used in this project. This scholarly project aims to improve the quality of end-of-life care amongst African Americans by assessing participants' awareness and knowledge about ADs, and improving modifiable behaviors associated with readiness to complete AD.

The behaviors include appointing an HCA, completing a living will or HCP, discussing wishes with loved ones and the physician.

Background

The factors that account for lower ACP amongst African Americans are more complex than often portrayed in the discussion. Laury, Greenle, and Meghani (2019) report that factors that affect African Americans' end-of-life care beyond trust include lack of access to care, lower income and education levels, relationships, and quality of communication with health care providers. The author's professional and personal experiences from bedside nursing and caring for a chronically ill parent have contributed to inquiries on the evidence related to the problem, possible interventions, and the best setting to achieve desired outcomes given the population involved.

Kwak and Harley (2005) reported that non-White ethnic groups generally lacked knowledge of ADs and were less likely to support it. ACP discussed when one's health care has deteriorated at the end-of-life remains difficult for patients and health professionals. The planning process tends to involve task-oriented documentation of crucial preferences such as resuscitation and place of death rather than discussing the patient's care goals (Pollock & Wilson, 2015). Koss and Baker (2017) report 40 percent of older adults in America become unable to make medical decisions at the end-of-life. The continuous progress with health care technologies in prolonging lives without necessarily improving quality of health, and the continuous gap in readiness for ACP, create the urgency for equitable health care and quality health care. When patients are admitted to the hospital in an acute or confused state without a pre-existing AD, there may be a delay in care (Carson & Bernacki, 2017). Further, the authors report health professionals understood the experiences that will take time to understand the patient's baseline knowledge of their health and end-of-life preferences from family members if there is access to one. If the health care professionals cannot find any history or care preferences for the patient in documentation, they may intuitively choose to do everything possible to save the patient's life. These decisions may be directed from individualized patient and family preferences. Sometimes, this may include a blood transfusion, an invasive surgical intervention, and resuscitation if the patient's heart stops. Carson and Bernacki (2017) report that the lack of AD planning may result in emotional distress in bereaved families, moral distress with health professionals, and escalated non-coursed costs without accompanying measurable benefits to patients' survival or quality of life end-of-life leave ethical confusion of what to do as the "right thing."

Although impeding factors like diagnosis, spirituality, and poverty are not modifiable by the nurse, the nurse plays a vital role in collaboration with health care and community partners to break barriers associated with the persistent gap in ACP decisions. For example, a stakeholder revealed that many people "shy" away from ACP conversations; they put it off later when they become sick because of uncertainties regarding the process and prioritize other stressful and more pressing things faced with often (personal communication, 2021). This procrastination partly explains why readiness for ACP may be lower in non-White or minority communities often dealing with different types of social and economic stressors. Building confidence with advance planning conversation is a juxtaposition based upon a voluntary discussion versus one that needed to occur to honor one's wishes during declining health prognosis.

Significance

Literature reports readiness for engagement in ACP follows expected behaviors reported in the process of AD completion and ACP itself (Fried, Redding, Robbins, Paiva, O'Leary, & Iannone, 2010). They said that these behaviors include completing a living will, HCP, communicating health care treatment preferences, perception of quantity versus quality of life with loved ones, and sharing these issues with the physician. The authors further report readiness is a process that occurs in stages and is affected by factors such as the individuals' values and understanding of what ACP means. Therefore, understanding the barriers to readiness for ACP will be helpful when proposing meaningful interventions to increase the completion of AD.

In a customer discovery process in a faith-based setting and as reported from initial interactions with the congregants on the topic of ACP, the DNP student determined a need to address the practice community gap based on non-compliance and knowledge of AD. The initial assessment data informed the project on impactful interventions that will meet the needs of the congregants based upon trust and the accurate information to make life-sustaining personal decisions. The hope is that individuals express improvement in any ACP behaviors (appoint an HCA, discuss wishes with loved ones and physicians, complete an HCP form) before the end of the project.

Problem Statement

Health and health care disparity among minority ethnic groups, especially African Americans, is a social and public health crisis that warrants mentioning when discussing the completion of AD. Furthermore, the combined impact of the Covid-19 pandemic, which disproportionately affected the Black individuals, and the police brutality against a Black American (Floyd, 2020), again exposed the effect of systemic racism on the well-being of African Americans. This project addresses equitable access to quality health care, and expert health care end-of-life discussion with licensed nursing professionals and their population (African American adults participants) was intended to improve ACP behaviors. The behaviors encompass making preferences known to loved ones and physicians and completing an AD.

Concepts and Definitions

ADs are treatment preferences and the designation of a surrogate decision-maker if an individual becomes incompetent to make medical decisions on their behalf, and AD may be categorized into three types, namely living will, power of attorney, and HCP (Davis, 2021). With the durable power of attorney for health care, the individual nominates one or more persons who will communicate their wishes or preferences should they become incapacitated.

A living will is a written statement that specifies the types of medical treatments an individual desires (Davis, 2021).

HCP is a legal document in which individuals select someone trustworthy to make health care decisions if they become incapable of making their wishes known (Davis, 2021).

Readiness describes the level of preparedness on one end of the spectrum (pre-contemplation phase) to contemplation, to taking action and to the other end, maintaining action on engaging in ACP. It should be noted that "readiness is not a linear process." This project focused on improving participants' behavior to identify and designate an HCA and to complete an HCP if possible.

PICOT Question

The purpose of this quality project is to seek an answer to the inquiry. Among African American congregants at a Christian Church in a suburban city in Massachusetts (P), is a multi-modal intervention (to include educational videos, print medium, and live discussions with participants) on advanced care planning (ACP) (I), over three months (T), associated with an increase in knowledge of ACP and readiness to identify an HCA and complete of Health Care Proxy (HCP) (O)?

Purpose Statement

Evidence suggests lower rates of ACP are associated with adverse health outcomes at end-of-life. Readiness in this project is the willingness to do something among the congregants. The ACP behaviors are the characteristic response identified in prior studies to complete an AD. They include appointing an HCA, informing family and physicians on choices and preferences, and completing an HCP. Improving ACP behaviors among the church-based participants may increase ACP and, as a result, improve rates of their AD completion and, subsequently, the cost of health care.

Impact of the Problem on a Population or System

The impact of ACP described in a study by Arruda, Abreu, Santana, and Sales (2019), identify patients who had ADs reported to have a lower rate of invasive interventions. These interventions included mechanical ventilation, artificial nutrition hemodialysis, cardiopulmonary resuscitation (CPR) maneuvers. They also said these patients experienced short hospital stays and death at home. Without ACP to direct health care professionals with preferred treatment options, patients lose their autonomy due to the complexity of their health care needs and time-sensitive decision-making. Individuals without AD may be subjected to costly, painful, and futile treatments that they may not have been chosen for themselves (Arruda, Abreu, Santana, & Sales, 2019).

Conversely, patients who completed advance directives during a time when decisions were part of a conversation with family and or health care provider, as compared to those who preferred heroic end-of-life care were more likely to be younger patients, non-Whites, and patients who were less likely to have health insurance (Garrido, Balboni, Maciejewski, Boa, & Prigerson, 2014). Thus, the factors that impede AD discussion and decision are varied and complex.

At the micro-systems level, the impact of one new ACP completed may mean a patient centered plan of care for that individual, which is directly linked to "comfort" at end-of-life (patient goals, regardless of what they are, are aligned with the treatment plans). Evidence suggests the impact of having an AD includes reducing caregiver stress, family feuds, and financial burden on the individual just as the health system. At a macro-systems level, the various systems need to think together to make meaningful change that is equitable for all patients. A process map linking Acute care, Primary care, and Community care may be a good place to start the collaboration work. Policies that recognize low ACP behaviors as a public health crisis, may encourage innovative practice-interventions that link the various systems and puts the patient at the center of the patient or community's care and health care system in general.

CHAPTER 2:

Literature Synthesis

Methods of Review

An electronic bibliographic search conducted in the CINAHL, MEDLINE Scholar databases, and Google Scholar website for the keywords; "Advance Care Planning," "African Americans," "readiness," and "faith-based" resulted in nine-hundred-and-sixty-six articles. The author performed data searches between May 2021 and December 2021. The inclusion criteria were peer-reviewed articles with publication dates from 2010 to 2021. Studies included ACP discussions, barriers to possessing advance directives, readiness for ACP, community interventions to increase enthusiasm for ACP. Some studies may have had led to hard searching expert opinions.

Exclusion criteria included articles written before 2010, written in a foreign language other than English and did not address interventions to increase AD completion, interventions targeted strictly in acute care settings. A total of one-hundred-and-fifty-four articles were screened. Following the exclusion criteria, one-hundred-and-thirty-two articles were further removed. The remaining twenty-two articles were screened for eligibility based upon criteria. Three articles were removed due to a small sample, having interventions designed for a foreign country and focusing on the dialysis patient population. Of the nineteen articles reviewed, fourteen had Level I evidence. Refer to the PRISMA diagram (Appendix G).

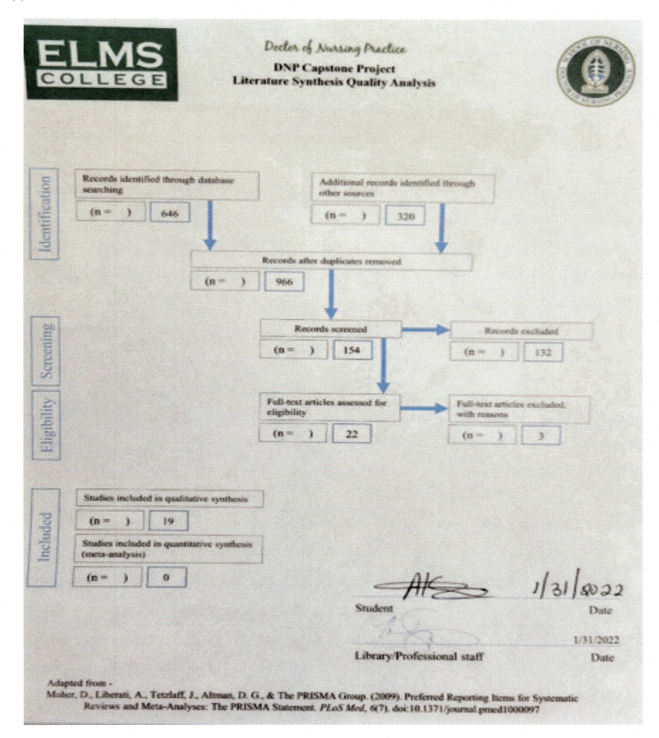

ELMS COLLEGE

Doctor of Nursing Practice
DNP Capstone Project
Literature Synthesis Quality Analysis

Identification

Records identified through database searching
(n =) 646

Additional records identified through other sources
(n =) 320

Records after duplicates removed
(n =) 966

Screening

Records screened
(n =) 154

Records excluded
(n =) 132

Eligibility

Full-text articles assessed for eligibility
(n =) 22

Full-text articles excluded, with reasons
(n =) 3

Included

Studies included in qualitative synthesis
(n =) 19

Studies included in quantitative synthesis (meta-analysis)
(n =) 0

Student _____ Date 1/31/2022

Library/Professional staff _____ Date 1/31/2022

Adapted from -
Moher, D., Liberati, A., Tetzlaff, J., Altman, D. G., & The PRISMA Group. (2009). Preferred Reporting Items for Systematic Reviews and Meta-Analyses: The PRISMA Statement. *PLoS Med*, 6(7). doi:10.1371/journal.pmed1000097

Appraisal of the Evidence

The review of evidence conducted by Huang, Neuheaus, and Chiong (2016), and Koss and Baker (2018), supports that African Americans are less likely to possess ADs and that 40 percent of older adults in America become unable to make medical decisions (Koss & Baker, 2017). In a nationwide study by Clark, Person, Gosline, and Block (2018), the evidence indicated racial differences in the designation of HCA, communication of goals, values, and preferences for end-of-life to health care providers' families. The result indicated that less than half of the one-thousand-eight-hundred-and-fifty-one participants had named an HCA, and only 14.5 percent of them ever had an end-of-life conversation with a health care provider. This QI project responds to the need to reduce the racial gap in ACP in the African American communities.

Most of the studies investigating possible contributory factors of AD possession reported that the HSB of the Black Americans were a significant factor. However, these studies were predominantly in medical and clinical settings and older adult patients during end-of-life care. In addition, ACP initiatives in community settings are limited (Pollock & Wilson, 2015; Herdeman & Karbeah, 2020) and were not often directed toward the affected population.

Miller (2018) wrote an integrated study of nineteen publications between 1990 and 2018 on nurses' and nursing students' knowledge and confidence regarding AD in Nursing Curricula. Fewer than half demonstrated knowledge or confidence regarding AD and that Nursing Programs that cover legal documents spend only 1.5 hours or less on AD. Six of twenty-two studies reviewed in this study shared that health professionals lack the knowledge and confidence to initiate and engage patients in ACP. While interventions to educate health care providers in clinical settings are ongoing, individuals in the community also need to be ready to begin ACP discussions with their health care providers for best outcomes.

Evidence suggests that ACP programs or interventions are often limited to the elderly population or at their end-of-life. The author extended this QI project to young adults (18 years) and adults with the rationale that accidents and acute illnesses that sometimes cause mental and physical disability may occur at any age. For example, in the three nationally famous cases involving Karen Ann Quinlan (1970s), Nancy Cruzan (1980s), and Terri Schiavo (1990s), they were all young women at the time, who were incapacitated due to the severity of their health status affecting their decision-making abilities, thus leaving the families and the courts to determine treatment plans for them. Also, Lance Armstrong was only twenty-five when he was diagnosed with cancer. Focusing on tailoring interventions that target older adults misses the opportunity to engage a sizable part of the population affected by a lack of readiness for ACP conversations.

The health care provider's role in the completion of AD is as essential as the role of the patient in this process because it often determines when conversations begin with the patient. Oskousi, Pandya, Weiner, Wong, Koch-Weser, and Ladin (2020) report only 7 percent of patients recalled being offered the opportunity to discuss issues about the capacity to engage in decision-making. Health care professionals in community settings usually do not need to initiate conversations about advance directives for various reasons, including time constraints and personal attitudes toward the subject. In addition, many patients present to the hospital without a pre-existing advance directive in acute states. Often, discussions of advance directives between health professionals and patients occur before the final days and weeks of life (Lakin, Koritsanszky, Cunningham, Maloney, Neal, Paladino, Palmor, Volgeli, Ferris, Block, Gawande, & Bernacki, 2017).

Discussion

The commonly reported assertion is that African Americans mistrust the health care system, contributing to limited, timely access to health care (Koss and Baker, 2017). Evidence suggests African Americans generally have "strong" cultural and religious ties to their communities. Therefore, it becomes imperative to explore reasons for ACP-hesitancy in the African American population and seek solutions to the possible causes of low ACP behaviors. These behaviors include identifying and naming an HCA or an HCP, discussing goals and preferences with health care providers and families, and completing an AD. If individuals and health care professionals are knowledgeable and skillful with the ACP process, there will be increased agency and readiness to become engaged in ACP programs and complete ADs. Additionally, these factors may contribute to a lack of action due to applicability to them.

The health-seeking behaviors (HSB) of African Americans are the most cited reason for the gap in ACP among Black patients. However, evidence suggests other elements have accounted for the status of ACP behaviors among African Americans. They include the physical, socio-cultural, economic, and psycho-spiritual factors.

Physical Factors with Advance Care Planning

The physical health status of individuals may influence whether and when they participate in ACP. For instance, patients diagnosed with cancer, kidney failure, heart disease, liver disease, and diabetes. Depending on the intensity of their symptoms, they may have had more opportunities in clinical settings and with family members to discuss advance directives. Evidence suggests that the sicker the patient is the more the urgency to make advance care directives (Oskoui, Pandya, Weiner, Wong, Koch-Weser, & Ladin, 2020).

Socio-Cultural and Economic Factors with Advance Care Planning

The age, sex, educational level, household income, marital status, values, and cultural norms of the patient may influence the possession of an AD. Older adults are more likely than younger individuals to have AD (Oskoui, Pandya, Weiner, Wong, Koch-Weser, & Ladin, 2020). White patients who are more educated, of higher household income, and marital status are more likely to have an AD than Black patients (Koss & Baker, 2017). Also, lived experiences and history of caring for others with chronic conditions may influence an individual's attitude toward ACP.

Oskoui, Pandya, Weiner, Wong, Koch-Weser, and Ladin (2020) reported that the most common reason for not completing advance directives was because some participants (18%) did not know what an AD was; meanwhile, 11 percent of them had not thought of completing one. For the 65 percent of participants who had an AD in their study, 32 percent stored theirs at home, 21percent said their family member kept it, 25 percent at the hospital, and only 7 percent indicated it was stored in a medical record. In addition, 45 percent of them indicated they were allowed to express their fears and concerns, and 42 percent indicated they had been informed that they could change their mind regarding their goals of care decision-making at any time. These findings support the argument that the issue of ACP, especially for Black patients, is complex and requires annual reviews to determine if there are behavioral changes. It informs this QI project, focusing on areas that may help center the interventions around the specific need of the affected population.

Health and health care disparity among minority ethnic groups, especially with African Americans, is a social facet worth mentioning with AD possession. Race remains a factor in health disparities. For instance, clinically speaking, the American Heart Association's (AHA) guideline for Heart Failure Risk Assessment predicts the risk of death in patients admitted to the hospital. Based on this risk screening tool, three additional points are assigned to non-Black patients, categorizing Black patients at a lower risk level (Vyas, Eisenstein, & Jones, 2020) and of which it is a known fact that African Americans have a higher risk of diabetes, kidney, and heart conditions when compared with White patients of White ethnic and racial groups. Because such instances are often underreported, it isn't easy to measure the degree.

Furthermore, the combined impact of the Covid-19 pandemic of 2020 (which disproportionately affected the Black population) and police brutality against a Black American (Flyod, 2020) refocused on the effect of systemic racism on Black individuals' well-being in America. To understand the disparity in ACP affecting the Black population, the author explored the concept of race as a contributory factor. Like any other public health crisis, ACP among African Americans requires system-thinking interventions to create long-term solutions and trust on the knowledge required to make an informed decision.

Psycho-Spiritual Element with Advance Care Planning

The familiar saying "mental health is healthcare" (author unknown) resonates by conjecture that, in traditional health care settings when a patient is deemed incompetent to make decisions due to their state of mental health. Someone else from the family or appointed by the courts will do so on the patient's behalf. If one is free of physical pain but has reported symptoms of a diagnosis of depression, they have impaired psycho-spiritual needs (Kolcaba, 2001). If one's faith prohibits them from talking about death, they may not want to discuss the AD-related topics leading to an informed decision. When individuals can manage their problems and pain, they enter a state of transcendence (Kolcaba, 2001) which is like a state of wholeness which surpasses every physical limitations.

Most African Americans believe in a god or a higher being from an insider's perspective. Their belief system may influence their attitude toward end-of-life care planning; a familiar narrative with African Americans is that "hope" is what keeps life going. As such, talking about the end-of-life with a family, say a parent, could upset the parent because it could be misinterpreted as loss of hope and or lack of compassion. One's belief system also depends on the level of acculturation for the African American. The lesser the level of acculturation, the more they hold on to their traditional values and beliefs. The lesser they may be eager to initiate conversations on the end-of-life vice versa.

For many African Americans who believe God is the Miracle Healer and the only one who has the power to take away life, they may resist engaging in AD discussions which indicate limiting life-sustaining treatments and hope for a healing miracle. Many of these practices guide their lifestyle which may also be culturally part of their value system. Johnson, Elbert-Avila, and Tusky (2005) report God is responsible for physical and spiritual health, and doctors are God's instrument. If a culture forbids end-of-life discussions and planning, it is less likely that the individual will initiate or participate in ACP discussions.

Faith leaders like pastors, priests, deacons, and elders are vital in Black communities as they have the community's trust and access to church members regularly. Therefore, this study aims at collaborating with church leaders from a faith-based community with a sizable population of African American backgrounds.

Environmental Factors with Advance Care Planning

Most of the evidence reviewed in this QI study had interventions to increase AD completion in medical settings. Although most of the studies cited that African Americans had lower odds of engaging in ACP discussions, this author could only locate one study which focused on the African American population. For this reason, the author broadened the people to include "Black Americans." This project responds to the critique that if any study seeks to inquire about racial inequality in care, the study should be community-led (Herdeman & Karbeah, 2020).

Possible Solutions

Best practices in discussing care goals include sharing prognostic information, eliciting decision-making preferences, understanding patients' fears and goals, and exploring tradeoffs and impaired function (Bernacki & Block, 2014). However, the ethnic variations in AD possession are not well understood. As a result, such interventions have not been highly successful despite the increasing interest in increasing prehospital advance care plans among black patients.

Van Scoy, Levi, Witt, Bramble, Richardson, Putzig, Levi, Wasserman, Chinchilli, Tucci, & Green (2020) used a low-cost conversation game to motivate underserved African Americans individuals to ACP. In the conversation game "Hello", individuals in groups of four to six participated in conversations related to ACP. As a result, after the intervention and within eleven months, ninety-one out of two-hundred-and-twenty participants (41%) of the individuals completed a new AD, one-hundred-and-seventy-six of two-hundred-and-twenty participants (80%) of the participants discussed end-of-life issues with their loved ones, 98 percent achieved at least one ACP behavior. This evidence informs the proposed community project of possible gains with ACP initiatives tailored to community settings and with the reference that such projects need to be community-led.

Cornally, McGlade, Weathers, Daly, Fitzgerald, O'Caoimh, Coffey, and Molloy (2015) described the 'Let ME Decide' Advance Care Planning (LMD-ACP) program which was developed and implemented in three long-term facilities to improve the quality of care at the end-of-life. The results showed enhanced care delivery and positive care environments for these homes. In addition, the Serious Illness Care Program was implemented as a structured training program for health care professionals at fourteen primary care clinics. As a result, patients in these participating clinics were more likely to engage in serious illness conversations than patients seen at the non-participating clinic (Lakin, Koritsanszky, Cunningham, Maloney, Neal, Paladino, Palmor, Volgeli, Ferris, Block, Gawande, & Bernacki, 2017).

Research studies indicate that ACP is necessary for individuals and even more so for people who have a chronic disease(s) and the elderly. For example, Levi, Simmons, and Green (2010) demonstrated that individuals with amyotrophic lateral sclerosis (ALS) could complete a computer-based decision aid for ACP and promote effective ACP. In addition, the Respecting Choices Program and the Providing End of life Advance Care Planning (PEACE program) for patients through education and evaluation of patients' preferences in the Primary Care setting (Cave, 2018) have been attempted with success when attempting to discuss this topic in the care setting.

Structured educational seminars with health care providers on ACP and communication with patients have been used in many studies to increase knowledge, attitude, and AD completion in medical settings. A systematic review conducted by Durbin, Fish, Bachman, and Smith (2010) indicated that combined written and verbal educational interventions were more effective than single written interventions in increasing the percentage of AD completion in an adult outpatient clinic and hospitalized elderly. To maximize desired outcomes for this project, the author appraised the multi-modal intervention as the best evidence practice model to improve ACP behaviors in participants.

Theoretical Model

Katherine Kolcaba's Comfort Theory (2001)

Nurses consciously and unconsciously use Katherine Kolcaba's Comfort Theory (2001) daily to promote patient comfort. Kolcaba distinguished three types of comfort: relief, ease, and transcendence, which occur in the physical, psycho-spiritual, environmental, and social contexts (Kolcaba, 2001).

Critical concepts in Kolcaba's Comfort Theory include health care needs, intervening variables, comfort, HSB, institutional integrity, best policies, best practices (Kolcaba, 2001). Important propositions to this framework translate from evidence-based practice (EBP) and are applicable in various practice settings. They included:

1. Nurses identify patients' comfort needs not met by the existing support system.

2. Nurses design interventions.

3. Intervening variables take into account agreed enhanced comfort and HSB.

4. If enhanced comfort is achieved, patients are empowered to participate in the HSB.

5. If patients engage in the HSB, nurses and patients become more satisfied in their health care.

6. When patients are satisfied with their health care in a specific institution that institution retains its integrity.

The Kolcaba Comfort Theory explains how comfort is the desired outcome of nursing care. The theory incorporated elements of the DNP project through the student-led implementation at the community church setting. As a result, the patient, or in the case of this project, is African American Congregants to be exposed to an educational awareness and knowledge of ACP discussions, which is intended to improve their ACP behaviors (such as appointing an HCA and completing an AD), ultimately increasing their personal comfort in the end-of-life discussions.

The Transtheoretical (TTM) Model, which was designed by Prochaska and DiClemente (1970), was incorporated with Kolcaba's Comfort Theory to best describe "readiness" in the process of ACP discussion and AD completion. The Transtheoretical Model has five stages or levels of change which can be measured and tracked from pre-contemplation, Preparation, Action, and Maintenance with ACP behaviors mentioned above. Increased readiness in, say, appointing an HCA or completing an HCP translates to increased comfort for the congregants during end-of-life, which is the overall goal of the QI project. How ready the congregants regarded ACP conversations, and AD completion was determined with the help of the "readiness scale" derived from the TTM model.

Conceptual Framework

The Plan-Do-Study-Act (PDSA) problem-solving conceptual model by Deming (2021) was applied to test the change in the intended outcome (improving ACP behaviors and AD completion) in this QI project. The author used the six dimensions of *The Institute of Medicine's Framework for Quality Healthcare*, an essential guide to ensuring the implemented project was within the standard practice (Agency for Healthcare Research and Quality 2018). It included safe, timely, effective, efficient, equitable, and patient-centered (STEEP). The current state of ACP for black individuals is *unsafe* when their wishes and preferences were not known; *ineffective* because bedside education is often too late.

In addition, *time* to treat the patient may impact health care professionals' decision-making as they wait for a directive in intervention from a family member or court-appointed, especially on complex care needs and decisions. Lastly, it is *not patient-centered* because the health care providers are not often aware of the patient's treatment preferences and wishes. The PDSA concept was suitable for this QI project because the first cycle (from planning the program, implementing interventions, assessing the impact of the implementation) to acting by conserving the gains made in the project while making modifications of interventions with subsequent cycles if applicable, to maximize best outcomes. It is thus a continuous process.

Goals and Objectives for the Project

The project's overall aim was to increase participants' awareness and knowledge about advance directives, improve modifiable behaviors of ACP, and determine the impact of an AD program on the perceived beliefs of the congregants in completing AD within three months period.

Goal 1: Increase the participants' knowledge of ACP during interactive educational sessions at the Church setting.

Objective one: To prepare basic educational materials on ACP and the process of completing a Health Care Proxy document.

Objective two: To disseminate the information to the participants in various modes (live discussions, prints, and educational videos) to increase knowledge and awareness on the ACP process.

Goal two: Determine if a multi-modal (live conversations, prints, and educational video) intervention increases readiness in modifiable ACP behavior in identifying and naming an HCA, discussing goals and preferences with health care providers and families, and completing the AD).

Objective one: To identify a readiness scale or tool to measure behavior change over the project implementation span.

Objective two: To administer a pre-discussion survey for baseline assessment of participants' level of ACP knowledge and behaviors and a post-discussion/intervention survey to measure the impact of the implementation of the multi-modal intervention.

Goal three: Increase the percentage of completed HCP (document), following the intervention.

Objective one: Initiate ACP conversations with the congregants in formal and informal ways as preferred and provide steps in completing the Massachusetts HCP form.

Objective two: Engage faith leaders and health care professionals in the community during implementation to sustain gains of the project and reinforce the ACP discussions.

Objective three: Provide a step-by-step guide in completing the Massachusetts Health Care Proxy document to participants who are ready to complete it.

CHAPTER 3:

Methodology

Context

Participants

Inclusion criteria for participation were congregants eighteen years and older who understand and write in English. Congregants under eighteen years of age spoke a different language, and those who did not wish to participate for any reason were permitted to leave.

The Setting, Population, and Sample Selection

The project was conducted in a faith-based community in Natick, Massachusetts. Membership ranged between ninety to one-hundred-and-thirty congregants annually, and over half of the congregants from 2019 identify as African Americans. Weekly Sunday attendance varied between thirty and fifty congregants in person and via zoom. The author used a convenience sample. Congregants who decided to remain in the Church premises after Church service were recruited after the consent was given and read. In addition, due to Covid-19 restrictions, some congregants attended the event via zoom. There were twenty-six participants in Session 1 and five participants in Session 2, bringing thirty-one participants in person and an unknown number of congregants via zoom. The author only collected data from participants present in person under the Elms Institutional Review IRB) Board requirement for this QI project plan.

Ethical Considerations

The ELMS IRB, on October 12, 2021, issued approval for the proposed QI project called "Honoring Your Choices," and the implementation phase began on October 17, 2022, and ended on December 12, 2022. The author did not use identifiers during data gathering and recording. For confidentiality, the data collected was stored in a locked password-protected computer and saved in a locked cabinet accessed only by the author.

The risk of harm to the congregants was minimized through voluntary participation, self-report questionnaires, de-identifying participants, and double lock to secure data gathered in a file accessed only by the author. In addition, participants were provided with the contact numbers for the Elms IRB and the Elms Capstone Specialist and Advisor to report any concerns they may have with the project implementation.

As the Project Manager, the author emailed guidelines that included a detailed description of the roles of the team partners. For instance, the Pastor a Stakeholder, made announcements about the project during services and was available for consultation and support if needed; the Clerk of the Session was in charge of forwarding flyers to the church's group email chain or projector. He was also the liaison for the project with the Session of the Church for updates. The author met with the Champion Nurse in the community in person and via email to ensure the nurse was comfortable with ACP discussions and that she understood her role. Finally, the author organized and delegated tasks to the appropriate team partners, allowing the author to focus on content and successful project implementation while protecting participants' rights.

Project Design and Methods

This QI study was a prospective quantitative design. However, a correlational design benefited the study because the aim of the study explored the relationship between nurses' intervention and the readiness of participants to engage in advanced ACP behaviors.

Prior Implementation

The readiness of this faith community's engagement in this QI project was assessed when the author accepted the invitation to the church's monthly session (board) meeting, attended by a Pastor, the Clerk of Session, Elders, and Deacons. The author described the purpose of the project. The board members all voted to permit the author to implement the project at the congregation. In addition, the Clerk of Session agreed to work closely with the author on the project.

The author received a written authorization or agreement from Project Site to complete the QI project (Appendix A). The author used a flyer to advertise the project (Appendix B) to the congregants through the church's newsletter called Hartford Happenings two weeks before the first date of the event. The Pastor and the Clerk of Session (Project Facilitator) acted as liaisons to the congregants. They facilitated creating awareness about the coming of this QI project by adding announcements on the "church-projector" during *Announcements* through the church group email. A week before the event's first session, the author announced to the congregation a brief description of the "Honoring Your Choices" project.

Appendix B: Advertisement Flyer for the QI Project

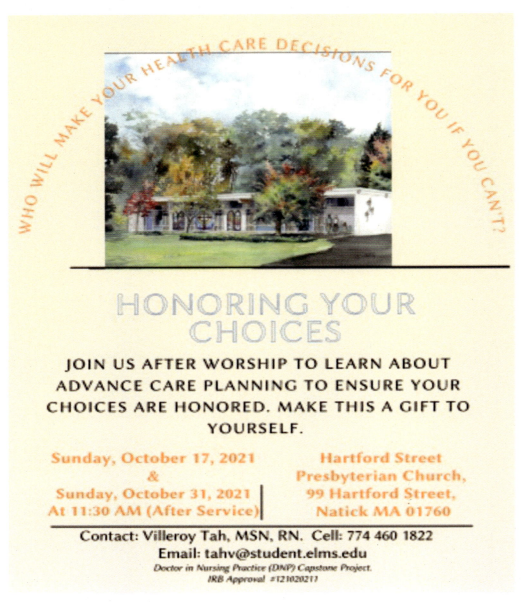

The author modified the Readiness Scale developed and validated by Fried, Redding, Robbins, Paiva, O'Leary, and Iannone (2010) to measure ACP knowledge, readiness to engage in ACP discussions, and rates of HCP completion amongst participants in the format of a questionnaire. The first eight items on the questionnaire measured readiness (Pre-contemplation, Contemplation, Action, and Maintenance) in ACP behaviors, including appointing an HCA, informing health providers and family members of goals and preferences, and completing ADs. Items 9 through 14 on the questionnaires were knowledge-based. Meanwhile, the pre-discussion survey only had additional three items (15–17): demographics (ethnicity, age group, and level of education). The last item on the post-discussion survey assessed the number of participants who have completed the HCP and when they completed it.

The author arranged print materials inside a two-bucket folder. The left pocket of the folder had the program advertisement flyer (Appendix B), the recruitment statement/consent (Appendix C), team members/contacts (Appendix D), and the pre-discussion survey (Appendix E). The middle part of the folder had "Facts" on ACP discussion tips and the educational video link (Appendix F) and "Prepare for Your Care" brochure (Appendix G). The right pocket of the folder had the Massachusetts Health Care Proxy (Appendix H), Advance Directive Notification Card (Appendix I), and the post-discussion survey (Appendix J). Each participant received a folder and a pen. The author used the organized folder to transition with content from the left, center, and to the right side of the folder.

See Appendix E: Pre-discussion survey.

During Implementation

On the day of the project event, the author introduced herself and the project team member(s) after the Church service. She briefly described the program's purpose and invited individuals interested in the program to remain seated while those who were not interested were excused to leave.

The author read the consent for participation. Next, the author counted the number of participants and distributed the program folders to each participant.

See Appendix C: Consent/Recruitment Statement.

Finally, the author provided instructions on completing the survey beginning with the pink-colored paper (pre-discussion survey) only, which took approximately five minutes. The goal of this survey was to assess baseline information for the participants before the discussions.

See Appendix E: Pre-discussion survey.

The author recorded content and then played a pre-recorded educational video (four-and-a-half minutes long) for congregants to watch and learn about basic information on ACP and the steps needed to appoint an HCA and to complete an AD.

Appendix F: Educational Video – Honoring your Choices

Open link below:

https://www.canva.com/design/DAEnxNbvceY/C_tU0sn_MnBnbG8kcFwjaQ/watch?utm_content=-DAEnxNbvceY&utm_campaign=designshare&utm_medium=link&utm_source=publishsharelink

Next, the author and a community nurse engaged in an open conversation with congregants on experiences with AD completion among individuals in the community. Finally, the author reviewed the "Prepare for Your Care" brochure, which highlights the five steps in ACP:

1. Choose a Medical Decision Maker

2. Decide what matters most in life

3. Choose flexibility for your decision-maker

4. Tell others about your wishes

5. Ask doctors the right questions

The author reviewed the Massachusetts Health Care Proxy form (Appendix H) with the participants.

Participants interested and ready completed the HPC document with the guidelines as reviewed voluntarily. Once completed, participants were told to make sure they gave a copy of their signed HCP to their Health Care Provider and informed the assigned HCA of their goals and wishes. Finally, the author gave directions on how to complete the wallet-sized Advance Directive Notification Card (Appendix I), which can be kept in the wallet behind the ID card for easy access during an emergency if ever needed.

See Appendix I: Advance Directive Wallet-Sized Notification Card.

The author requested that the green-colored post-discussion survey (Appendix J) be completed, taking four minutes. The author collected the surveys and placed them in a locked box only accessible to the author. The approximate time spent on the event was an hour from when Church service was concluded. Next, the author announced that another session of the event was scheduled in two weeks for individuals who could not attend or wish to attend the program again

Post-Implementation

The author who was the project leader remained available to the congregants who asked questions in person, telephone, and by email. The author reminded the congregants that although the project was closed, the team members were still available to answer questions and help with ACP and AD completion if needed. Finally, the author sent a closing notification to the project site (Appendix L) and to the Elms IRB (Appendix M), which officially ended the *Honoring Your Choices* project.

Method of Evaluation

Identifying three common behavioral characteristics of ACP concepts was key to beginning measurement development. How ready participants were engaged in identifying an HCA, discussing goals and preferences with health care providers and families, and completing HCP was measured using the staging algorithms. For instance, if a participant answered "yes" to the question "Do you have an HCA?", the participant would need to indicate if they appointed an HCP six months ago (in the Maintenance phase) or they did today (Action phase). If they have not thought about assigning an HCP, they were in the Pre-Contemplation phase. If a participant is thinking about appointing an HCP, they are in the Contemplation phase. A review of the aggregate responses on phases the participants was at pre-intervention and after the intervention informed the readiness state of the participants.

Data Management and Security

Data collected on the questionnaires was entered in a password-locked computer, accessible only to the author and destroyed three years later.

Methods of Analysis

The author used an Excel spreadsheet to enter the raw data from each participant on each survey item. Then, each item on the Pre-Discussion survey was analyzed and compared against Post-Discussion Survey items and presented on tables and charts (Table 3).

Data Collection Tools or Instruments

Data collected was self-reported on two color-coded survey documents (orange for the pre- and green for the post-survey) on the paper and the survey had components of the Likert Scale. Questions 9, 10, 11, 13, and 14 were dichotomous (Agree or Disagree). The rest of the questions had three to four responses for the participant to select the most applicable option.

The goals of the QI project were to increase awareness and knowledge about ACP, improve readiness to engage in ACP behaviors, and determine the effectiveness of an advanced directive program in a community setting that can improve AD completion. To evaluate if the program effectively increased awareness and knowledge of ACP, the author used the aggregate responses from the pre- and post-surveys to compare baseline data from answers provided after the nursing intervention.

To measure readiness in ACP behaviors (appointing an HCA, informing others of their choices, and completing an HCP), the author incorporated elements of a validated tool, the Readiness scale algorithm by Fried, Redding, Robbins, Paiva, O'Leary, and Iannone (2010).

Item 15 on the post-intervention survey was used to assess the program's effectiveness at improving AD completion.

Sustainability Considerations

The Clerk of Session, who acted in the role of Project Facilitator, is also involved in other church committees. The Champion Nurse lives and is familiar with most African American congregants in the church. And the Mental Health Counselor is a long-standing member of the church. The pastor, who is passionate about social justice calls, has inquired about extending the program to the Co-Habitant Portuguese Church sharing the same building. With the program's closing, congregants still have access to all these team members who have agreed to support, in one way or the other, the Congregants on ACP-related discussions.

Project Timeline

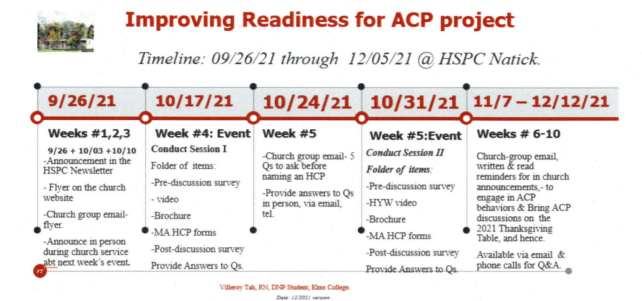

Improving Readiness for ACP project

Timeline: 09/26/21 through 12/05/21 @ HSPC Natick.

9/26/21	10/17/21	10/24/21	10/31/21	11/7 – 12/12/21
Weeks #1,2,3	**Week #4: Event**	**Week #5**	**Week #5:Event**	**Weeks # 6-10**
9/26 + 10/03 +10/10 -Announcement in the HSPC Newsletter	Conduct Session I Folder of items:	-Church group email- 5 Qs to ask before naming an HCP	*Conduct Session II* *Folder of items:*	Church-group email, written & read reminders for in church announcements,- to engage in ACP behaviors & Bring ACP discussions on the 2021 Thanksgiving Table, and hence.
- Flyer on the church website	-Pre-discussion survey - video	-Provide answers to Qs in person, via email, tel.	-Pre-discussion survey -HYW video	
-Church group email- flyer.	-Brochure -MA HCP forms		-Brochure -MA HCP forms	
-Announce in person during church service abt next week's event.	-Post-discussion survey Provide Answers to Qs.		-Post-discussion survey Provide Answers to Qs.	Available via email & phone calls for Q&A.

Villeroy Tah, RN, DNP Student, Elms College.

Date: 12/2021 version.

Resources/Budget

The estimated price points for items used to complete this project included: a Notebook journal for writing notes in real-time during the intervention phase ($10), a locked box to secure paper surveys and data gathered ($50), printing paper and ink for hard copy surveys, brochures, and flyers ($120), one hundred pens ($20) to complete surveys, customized decorative balloons ($30), small bottles of hand sanitizers-giveaways ($40), and a computer for data recording ($350). The estimated cost assessed by the author was $610. Team members participated in the project voluntarily without pay.

Photo of some participants on the first day of program implementation (shared with consent).

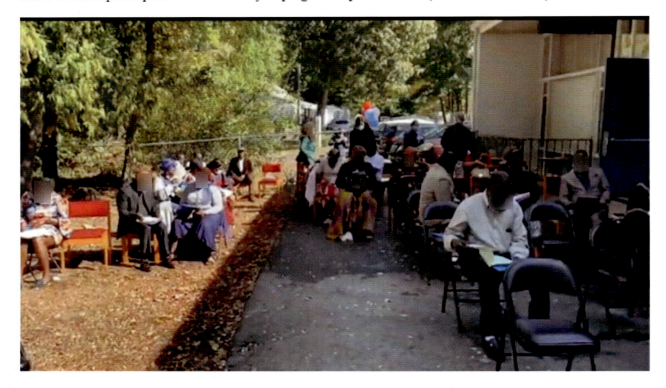

CHAPTER 4:

Project Results

Results

This QI project aims at initiating ACP discussions in the community to increase ACP behaviors like identifying an HCP and completing ADs. The survey was completed by thirty-one participants on a single site on two separate days, two weeks apart. One respondent was excluded due to a missing post-discussion survey. The final sample was thirty.

Description of Sample/Population

Thirty-two percent (10) of the participants were in the age group forty-nine to fifty-eight years, 22 percent (7) in the thirty-nine to forty-eight age group, 16 percent (5) participants in the twenty-nine to thirty-eight age group, 13 percent (4) participants in the fifty-nine to sixty-eight age group, 9.7 percent (3) in the sixty-nine to seventy-eight age group, and 3.2 percent (1) participant in the eighteen to twenty-eight age group. The table below is an illustration of the sample population in percentages.

Table 1: Demographics

Demographics	Number (#) of Participants	# of Participants in Percentages
Ethnicity		
1. Black	26	83%
2. White	3	9.6%
3. Others	2	6.4%
Age		
1. 18 – 28	1	3.2%
2. 29 – 38	5	16.1%
3. 39 -48	7	22.6%
4. 49 – 58	10	32.2%
5. 59 – 68	4	13%
6. 69 – 78	3	9.7%
7. 79 – 88	0	0
8. 89 - above	0	0
Highest Level of Education		
1. High School or Less	7	22.6%
2. More than High School	23	74.2%
3. No Response	1	3.2%

Forty-eight percent (15) of participants indicated in the pre-intervention survey, question 1, that they had appointed an HCP, while 37 percent (11) participants indicated they had appointed an HCP. When asked during pre-intervention how long ago the participant(s) appointed an HCP if applicable, 6.7 percent (2) participants indicated "Within the past six months," 42 percent (13) of participants said, "More than six months ago," while 52 percent (16) participants indicated "Not applicable." In the post-intervention survey,

13 percent (4) participants indicated "Within the past six months," 43 percent (13) participants indicated "More than six months ago" while 43 percent (13) participants indicated "Not applicable."

Project Outcomes

In question three, participants were asked, "Which of the following types of Advance Directive(s) do you have?" Pre-intervention survey, 20 percent (6) of participants indicated that they had a living will, 3 percent (1) indicated they had the Durable Power of Attorney, 22.5 percent (7) indicated they had an HCP, 10 percent (3) indicated they had health insurance, 3 percent (1) indicated "still reflecting," 6.5 percent (2) indicated they did not need an HCP, and 10 percent (3) did not respond to the question. Contrary at post-intervention, 13 percent (4) participants indicated they had the living will, 6.7 percent (2) indicated they had the Durable Power of Attorney, 50 percent (15) had the HCP, 3 percent (1) indicated "still reflecting," 3 percent (1) participant indicated they did not need an AD, while 10 percent (3) had more than one type of AD. See Figure 1 below.

Figure 1: Pre and Post Intervention Assessment on the types of Advance Directives possessed by participants

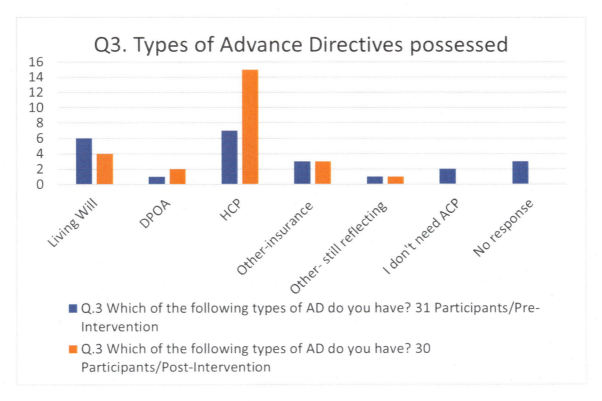

Question four was a follow-up from question three (how long ago did you complete the Advance Directive indicated in question three?). At the pre-intervention survey, 13 percent (4) of participants indicated they completed an AD "Within the past six months"; 50 percent (15) of participants said, "More than six months ago"; 6.4 percent (2) of participants indicated they were "uncomfortable to think about Advance Directives," and 10 percent (3) indicated they did not need it, while 27 percent (8) of participants did not respond to the question. At post-intervention, 22.5 percent (7) indicated they completed the advance directive "Within the past six months"; 45 percent (14) more than six months ago, 3 percent (1) indicated they were uncomfortable, 10 percent (3) did not need it, while 13 percent (4) participants did not respond to the question.

In Question five, participants were asked if they had already communicated with family or friends about prolonged-life treatments. Thirty-three percent (10) of participants indicated "Yes," while 67 percent (20) of participants indicated "No" they have not communicated with their family or friends. When asked how long ago they spoke with family or friends (question six), 30 percent (10) of participants indicated "More than six months ago," 3 percent (1) of participants indicated "Within the past six months," while 63 percent (19) did not respond to the question.

In Question seven, participants were asked, "Have you communicated with your doctor about what was is important to you?" Twenty-seven percent (8) participants indicated "Yes, I have," 73 percent (23) indicated "No, I haven't," and 3 percent (1) indicated "No, I am uncomfortable." When asked how long ago they communicated what was important to them with the doctor, 7 percent (2) participants indicated "Within the past six months, 20 percent (6) indicated "More than six months ago," while 77 percent (23) of participants indicated "Not applicable."

Questions 9 through 14 were knowledge-based, in the dichotomous structure. Details on the questions and responses at pre-intervention versus responses at post-intervention is presented below. Table 2 represents the Pre- and Post-Knowledge-based assessment by the questioning specific knowledge understanding.

Table 2: Pre and Post Intervention - HCP Knowledge-based (questions 9, 10, 11, 13 and 14)

	Survey Questions	Pre-Intervention (n = 30)			Post – Intervention (n = 31)		
	Questions	Agree	Disagree	No Response	Agree	Disagree	No Response
Q9.	I have the right to refuse medical treatment	80.6% (25)	19.4% (6)	0	83.3% (25)	17% (5)	0
Q10.	An HCP is someone who would make decisions on my behalf should…	80.6% (25)	16% (5)	3.2% (1)	83.3% (25)	10% (3)	6.7% (2)
Q11.	Once I sign an HCP, it cannot be changed	16% (5)	74% (23)	9.7% (3)	6.7% (2)	86.7% (26)	6.7% (2)
Q13.	An HCP is legal if only drawn up by a lawyer	6.5% (2)	90% (27)	6.5% (2)	6.7% (2)	86.7% (26)	6.7% (2)
Q14.	If I talked to my doctor, I don't need to talk to my family about my choices…	3.2% (1)	93.5% (29)	3.2% (1)	3.2% (1)	90% (27)	6.7% (2)

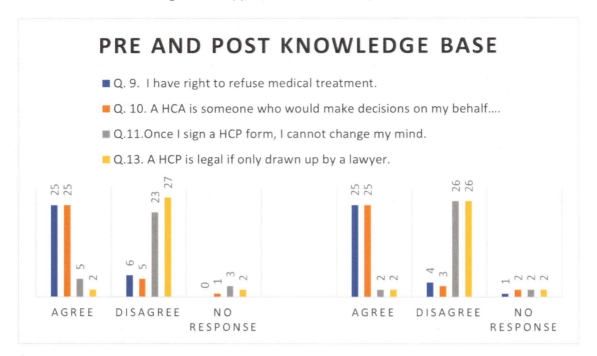

Participants were asked in question 12, "Where is it important to keep a copy of your HCP?" The response required the participants selects all appropriate choices (At Home, With my doctor, With a Family member, and All of the Above). At pre-intervention, 16 percent (5) participants indicated they would keep a copy of the HCP with a family member, 80.5 percent (25) participants indicated "Al of the Above," while 3.2 percent (1) had other combinations. During post-intervention, 6.7 percent (2) participants indicated they would keep a copy of HCP with a family member, 90 percent (27) indicated "All of the above," and 3 percent (1) participants chose with the doctor and a family member.

Description of the Data/Results

Lastly, 23 percent (7) participants indicated at the end of the project that they completed a new HCP during the program implementation: 23 percent (7) of participants indicated they would complete an HCP within the next three months, 33 percent (10) indicated they would in the next six months, 7 percent (2) of the participants did not plan on completing an HCP, 3 percent (1) participant indicated they already had one, and 10 percent (3) of participants did not respond to the question. Figure 3 pictorially describes the status of Participants on the Health Care Proxy completion.

Figure 3. Status of Participants on HCP Completion

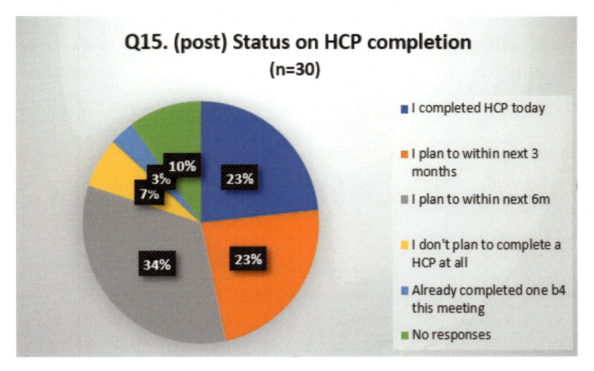

The author assessed the level of education (High School or Less and More than High School) against questions 1, 5, 7, 11, and 16. Sixty percent (3 out of 5) of participants who had indicated they had not appointed a HCA had a High School or Less educational status. In contrast, 31 percent (5 out of 16) of participants who indicated they had appointed a HCA had More than High School level.

In Question five, 30 percent (3 out of 10) of participants who indicated they had communicated their goals with family were those of the High School and More or Less than High School status, while 70 percent (7 out of 10) were from the More than High School group.

In Question seven, 37.5 percent (3 out of 8) of participants who indicated they had communicated what was important to them with the doctor were those of the High School or Less than High School group, while 62.5 (5 out of 8) had High School and More education.

In Question 11, 17 percent (4 out of 23) of participants who indicated "Disagree" to the statement that once signed, an HCP cannot be changed were of Less than High School educational group. In comparison, 83 percent (19 out of 23) of participants who indicated "Disagree" had More than High School status. There were 23 percent (7) participants in the age groups forty-nine to sixty-eight who had High School or Less level.

In the age group 18–38, 23 percent (7) of participants had Less than High School status. In responding to question five, 20 percent (2 out of 10) of participants in this age group who indicated they had communicated their goals with family members were of whom Less than High School group, while 80 percent were of the More than High School level. Twenty-five percent (2 out of 8) participants who indicated they had communicated what was important to the doctor were of High School or Less group, while 75 percent (6 out of 8) were from the More than High School group. On question 11, 26 percent (6 out of 23) of participants who "Disagree" with the statement that an HCP cannot be changed once signed were of the High School or Less group. Meanwhile, 74 percent (17 out of 23) participants who indicated "Disagree" were of the More than High School group. Of this age group, 100 percent (7 out of 7) of participants who indicated "All the Above" option on question 12 were those of the More than High School group.

Fifty-seven percent of participants were in the age group(s) thirty-nine to fifty-eight. In this age group, 61 percent (14 out of 23) participants had More than High School educational levels. In Question one, 39 percent (9 out of 23) of participants in the age group thirty-nine to fifty-eight indicated they had appointed an HCA; 40 percent (4 out of 10) of participants indicated they had communicated their goals with family, and 37.5 percent (3 out of 8) indicated they communicated what was important to the doctor. In Question 11, 48 percent (11 out of 23) of participants "Disagree" with the statement that once signed, an HCP cannot be changed. In comparison, 56 percent (14 out of 25) of participants on question 12, indicated the "All the Above" option when asked where it is important to keep a copy of the HCP.

Twenty-three percent (7) of participants were in the fifty-nine to seventy-eight age group. Seventy-one percent (5 out of 7) of participants in this group were of the High School or lower educational level. In question one, 31 percent (5 out of 16) of participants in this age group indicated they had appointed an HCA, 40 percent (4 out of 10) of participants indicated they had communicated their goals with family members (question 5), and 37.5 percent (3 out of 8) of the participants indicated they had communicated what was important to them to the doctor (question 7). In question 11, 17 percent (4 out of 23) of these participants indicated they "Disagree" with the statement that an HCP cannot be changed once signed. Lastly, in question 12, 20 percent (5 out of 25) of participants indicated the "All of the Above" option when asked important places to keep a copy of the HCP.

CHAPTER 5:

Evaluation

The level of Readiness to engage in ACP behaviors, especially completing the Advance Directive, was facilitated by incorporating the five elements of the Transtheoretical Model (TTM) in the data collection survey. Pre-contemplation meant "over six months," Contemplation meant "within six months," Action meant "within three months," and Maintenance meant "over one year." Twenty-three percent of participants stated they completed a new Health Care Proxy document during the program, Fifty-seven percent of participants indicated that they planned on completing an HCP within the next three months (23%) to six (34%) months Per the readiness scale, this translates to 23% in the Action phase, 23% in the pre-contemplation phase, and 34% of participants were in the contemplation phase when completing Advance Directives.

Although a higher number of participants had indicated at the beginning of the project that they had an Advance Directive, when asked to name the type of AD they had, 3 (10%) of participants documented they had health insurance, and 1 Participant said they had a Life Insurance. It became clear there was a gap in knowledge on Advance Directive and its various types. A participant stated they did not need an AD.

A myth about ACP and AD completion from the evidence was that it could not be changed once they complete an Advance Directive. There was no correlation between the level of education and Item 11 on the Survey (once signed, preferences cannot be changed). Thirty percent of participants did not answer the question correctly.

Outcomes

Evidence suggests that advance care planning and Advance Directive completion are indicators of comfort and quality care at the end of life. In addition, individuals who have a completed AD in their medical records have increased opportunities for their care to be centered on their care goals, choices, and treatment preferences because the health care team honors those choices in the plan of care for the individual. This DNP led QI project was aimed at improving ACP behaviors among African Americans in the community. They are reported to have lower odds of having ACP discussions and AD completion when compared to their white counterparts.

Findings in response to the goals established at the outset of this project included:

The first goal was to initiate ACP conversations intended to increase awareness and knowledge of the ACP process and activities. This objective was met as evidenced by a comparison of post-discussion survey responses from the pre-discussion responses. For instance, there was a 13% change in participants who became aware of the fact that they could change their minds after signing a Health Care Proxy. Also, there were mixed responses on where completed Health Care Proxy should be kept. While some thought it should be kept at home. A completed ACP document on a patient's bookshelf is useless if a copy is not shared with the doctor and family members.

The second goal was to use a multi-modal (live discussion, prints, and educational videos) intervention approach to increase Readiness in ACB behaviors (identifying a Health Care Agent, communicating goals with Health Care Providers and families, and completing AD if ready). This goal was met as 47% of participants indicated at least one ACP behavior they were active in at the end of the program. That is participants who reported they newly completed an HCP (23%), spoke with their health care provider (7%), and spoke with family members (17%) about what was important to them during the implementation of the project. Unfortunately, the implementation time was not long enough to allow the author to gather data specific to those who were able to meet with Health Care Providers to have these discussions with them. However, others indicated they named an HCP and discussed it with family members.

The last goal was to assess if the designed project effectively improved Advance Directive Completion. This objective was met as 23% of participants indicated they completed a new Health care Proxy during this project and 57% of participants said they would be completing the HCP within three to six months.

Resources and Budget impact

Having a community-led QI project like "Honoring Your Choices" was cost-effective in that the personnel who were involved in the project were identified community members with the required skills needed, and therefore, there was no need for hiring team members. The Pastor and the Clerk of the Session were readily available as the Healthcare Professionals in the community were. The cost incurred directly went into printing documents, buying pens and small bottles of hand sanitizers to ensure infection control guidelines were followed to prevent a covid19 infection outbreak.

Evaluation of the Theoretical Framework

Kolcaba's Comfort Theory was incorporated as demonstrated with key drivers pertinent to the African American population for this QI project. In addition, the author's or theorist's integrated framework called the *Collaborative Cultural Competence (C3) in Advance Care Planning,* was designed specifically to the project's needs.

The assumptions determined: (1) That Individuals' physical and psycho-spiritual health determines the degree of patients' needs, (2) That individuals may have different family members assigned by norm in their culture for effective decision making, including health care decisions, (3) that Family Health Care decision-makers may not need to be informed that they are Health Care Agents-they presume the role, (4) the Nurse and the health care providers must be culturally competent to meet the individual's needs, (5) that Gatekeepers in the community are essential influencers in individual's health care planning, (6) Collaboration with gatekeepers and healthcare professionals in the community builds trust, (7) when outcomes are positive, individuals trusts the institution, (8) All these complex variables contribute to a positive health-seeking behavior (HSB) (9) these positive HSB enhances comfort with rewards the positive behavior. See Figure 4 below.

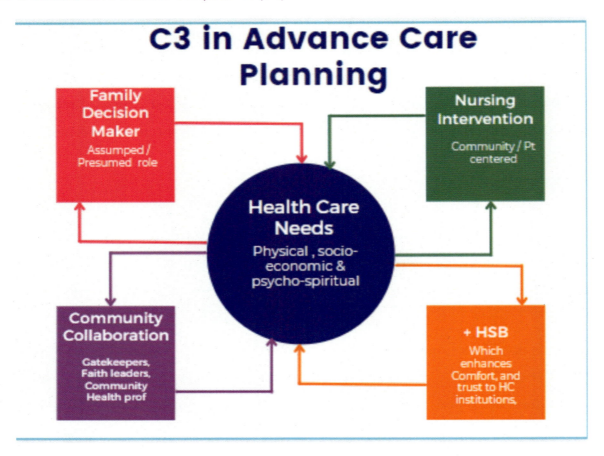

The concepts used in the C3 in the ACP model guided the author to identify and describe the factors that may be accounting for ongoing issues with ACP discussions and AD completion amongst African Americans, and design interventions and the variables which accounted for enhanced ACP behaviors. With the understanding that owning an AD ensures comfort at end-of-life, the participants learned and enagegd to become empowered in ACP discussions and complete AD if ready. Incorporating the TTM was appropriate to understanding where the participants were at the beginning versus the end of the project. The concept map used (PDSA) is most suitable to continue with the project's gains and make changes over the following cycles as informed by the first cycle of implementation.

Strengths and Limitations of the Project

The design of this QI project involved formal and informal discussions with the participants on advance care planning and the process of completing a health care proxy (HCP). Although outcome measures were gathered via the Pre and Post discussion surveys, anecdotal feedback received through in-person conversations and emails informed the author of other complexities or barriers to ACP discussions and AD completion among participants. The following were statements made by three participants to the author during the implementation of the project:

> *"Thank you for bringing this conversation to us. When I was made the HCA for my sick aunty, some of my family members were very upset with me for acting in that role because I was not the Successor (Head of Household)".*

> *"Thank you for opening our eyes; we needed it!"*

> *"It gets pushed off more pressing things, and then we procrastinate about getting it done."*

> *"I had this conversation with my doctor; it was a difficult one."*

This feedback supports the need for more studies in this population to understand the role of the head of households in ACP discussions and AD completion among African Americans and other possible barriers. Secondly, partnering with a community nurse and a mental health worker from the congregation was an asset to the project. They became support and contacts for any Congregant who may have questions or need additional help with ADC and AD completion. Another strength of the project was getting the Gatekeepers involved. While the Clerk of Session acted as a liaison between the church's ruling body (Session), the Congregants, and the Project Team Members, the Pastor was available as a Spiritual Counselor to any participant who may need it. This collaboration with the faith leaders was probably why the project was well received.

Limitations of the project included restrictions posed by the Covid-19 pandemic. The QI project was introduced when churches were re-opening from the second lockdown. About 90% of the congregants were attending services via Zoom, and the indoor capacity was limited to ten persons for indoor events. The author navigated this limitation by advertising the project with a flyer via the church›s newsletter, group email, church projector, and in-person discussions three weeks before the first scheduled event. The event was moved outdoors following Covid-19 restriction guidelines. Online participants were excluded from this sample even though they participated in the discussions because the proposed project plan limited the author to collect hard copy surveys.

The prospective design may have limitations. The author's active presence during discussions and data recording to observe the impact of exposure (Indeed Editorial Team, 2021) may have influenced participants' responses. The Hawthorne Effect is a likely limitation, a phenomenon identified with unwitting confounding variables under a study by itself to show behavioral changes due to an awareness of being observed (Wickstrom, and Bendix, 2000). Although not deemed research by the ELMS IRB, this quality improvement study conducted during the pandemic mandates in Massachusetts with appropriate social distancing for public health reasons engaged the congregation with the inclusive presence of the author. For this limitation, the participants were aware to direct their questions to the project leader and other project team members they may feel comfortable to speak about the topic, and not be well-known to them. The project team provided support and encouragement in addition to the focus of why the project was conducted at the setting.

The sample size (n=30) as the identified population of the study. Although the sample was sufficient for a quality improvement project, it is not enough to make the outcome generalizable as to the African American Population. For a larger sample in the future, more churches should be invited to participate in the project and recruitment of more congregants to the educational session after service.

Another limitation was limited research studies were conducted with the African American population. As a result, most of the studies used the umbrella term "Black" to describe their sample population. It is vital to note essential cultural differences with blacks of African descent.

The author created the Pre- and Post-intervention surveys by incorporating concepts and questions from the validated Readiness Scale by Fried, Redding, Robbin, Paiva, O'Leary, and Iannone (2010) to collect data from Participants. However, the author is a novice and not an expert in tool development.

Lastly, the implementation time was not long enough for the author to follow up with participants who may decide to speak to their health care providers about their wishes and treatment preferences. That is, it may take a few weeks to months to have a wellness visit appointment scheduled with the Health Care Provider, thereby, making it difficult to determine actual behavior change from this QI project. There was also limited time for Participants to sufficiently engage with their family members to discuss what was important to them and appoint Health Care Proxies. A Post-intervention check-in session after a few weeks of the intervention, may provide more insight on the impact of the project on ACP behaviors.

Plans for dissemination of the project

The author plans to disseminate the project results in an oral presentation at Elms College on Scholarship Day. The results will also be shared with the congregation through a poster presentation. An in-person presentation or online Poster presentation will be done. The author is exploring options to publish the project results in the Journal of Nursing Quality (JNQ) which focuses on publishing QI studies. The hope is that the gains from this project will be shared and replicated for improvement in health outcomes and health systems.

Implications for Future Practice

A systems approach to Advance Care Planning (ACP) and AD completion may benefit patients and other stakeholders, including collaboration between Public Health Agencies, Faith-Based Organizations, Medicare and Medicaid programs, Home Care Agencies, Nursing Home Consortiums, and Primary Care Practices. Although progress in this area was made under the health reform bill under Obama Care in 2009 and the Medicare reimbursement bill of 2016, more would have been accomplished if the communities directly affected were engaged in the interventions. The benefit of such collaboration will be helpful when other public health crises like vaccine hesitancy remain high in specific ethnic and patient populations. Unfortunately, current policies do not translate easily into non-clinical practices.

Clinical care and policy should recognize the variety most of the studies found and used to review the evidence for this project were done in the Black American population. There are noticeable variations in the African American and Black American communities that may need to be considered when tailoring community-centered or patient interventions. Clinical care and policy should recognize the various values and preferences found among diverse racial and ethnic groups (Kwak & Haley, 2005).

DNP Essentials

The increased legislature and health policies are needed to resolve or close healthcare access gaps. The recent move in Massachusetts to have Nurse Practitioners practice as independent practitioners is a step forward in recognizing the profession of nursing as a part of the solution to the public health crisis. It becomes vital to support the public health infrastructures and utilize systems thinking approaches with interventions. It is also essential to operationalize elements of a project as this one to ensure the outcomes based upon the project goals may be met during a reasonable timeframe to educate and inform participants as well as to measure if the impact of this type of project would elicit more complete AND forms.

The American Association of Colleges of Nurses (AACN, 2006) laid principles called "Essentials" of Doctoral Education for advanced nursing practice to meet the demands of the changing healthcare landscape. The focused practice principles include:

1. Nursing science and theory; scientific underpinnings for practice

2. Systems thinking, healthcare organizations, and the Advanced Practice Nurse

3. Clinical scholarship and evidence-based practice

4. Information systems/technology and patient care technology for the improvement and transformation of health care

5. Healthcare policy for advocacy in healthcare

6. Interprofessional collaboration for improving patient and population health outcomes

7. Clinical prevention and population health for improving the Nation's health

8. Advanced Nursing Practice

According to the AANC, the DPN graduate is equipped to design, influence, and implement health care policies and advocate for healthcare policies that address social justice and health equity issues. Since these Essentials laid the foundation for the DNP degree, the degree to which DNP faculty and students incorporate them into their Capstone projects is not known. Garritano, Glazer, Willmarth-Stec (2016) reported a moderate number of articles that disseminated DNP capstone project findings. The authors indicated that the results fell short of showing which DNP Essentials were used in the projects. Recommendations from the AACN do not oblige students to use all the Essentials in a project. This section describes how this author incorporated the eight DNP Essentials in this quality improvement project.

Essential I: Scientific Underpinnings for Practice. Firstly, the author used the body of knowledge from literature searches, appraised it, and presented it to the Elms Capstone experts and peers on the PICO question. This essential helped provide historical context to facts and data, which informed the author of design and interventions based on current information. Then, with the motivation from Katherine Kolcaba's Comfort theory, the author incorporated relatable concepts to describe the issues and the process of resolving the identified problem of low advance directive completion among African Americans. The author created an assessment tool to evaluate baseline behavior with Advance Care Planning based upon evidence translated from research studies and practice knowledge. The scientific method revealed small ecosystems, which may yield positive outcomes given collaboration and cultural sensitivity among stakeholders involved. Collaborative Cultural Competence (C3) in Advance Care Planning is thus a suggested model derived from this essential.

Essential II: Organizational and Systems Leadership for Quality Improvement and Systems Thinking. The author assumed the role of a transformational leader by organizing meetings with stakeholders to explore existing structures and resources. The author used cost-effective strategies like utilizing available resources (health care professionals in the community and faith leaders) to safely meet the affected population's needs. The author designed, implemented, and evaluated evidence-based interventions from Nursing and other Sciences. For instance, the evidence that a multimodal approach was more effective at chancing Advance Care Planning behaviors was a key consideration when planning and implementing the project.

Essential III: Clinical Scholarship and Analytical Methods for Evidence-Based Practice.

The author linked clinical scholarship and evidence-based practice by operationalizing the systems to create a patient-centered intervention. The implementation of the QI project in the community setting was intended to meet the affected population at their baseline. The author used prior experience from caring for patients at the bedside, with knowledge gained in doctoral study to identify the ACP gap in the African American population. Finally, the author used the following scholarship activities; development of the DNP proposal, collecting and evaluating data, writing the manuscript, and preparing to disseminate the findings to internal and external stakeholders and public health experts.

Essential IV: Information Systems/Technology and Patient Care Technology for the Improvement and Transformation of Health Care. The author used information and technology systems to design advertisement flyers, brochures, and educational videos, made available in hard copies and via a link.Much of the evidence was identified through electronic bibliography databases found in the literature searches.

Essential V: Health Care Policy for Advocacy in Health Care. This Essential prepares the DNP student in advocacy work at various levels (Garitano, Glazer, Willmarth-Stec, 2016). The author analyzed health care policies that have facilitated Advance Directive Completion with the findings, showing a general increase in AD completion with a continuous gap among African Americans. Then, the author participated in the Clinical site (Session) Committee meeting when accessing the need of the Congregants. The author met with Gatekeepers of the community and advocated for collaboration to increase ACP readiness and engagement among the affected population. The author did this by developing a network of Stakeholders (e.g., Faith leaders, Health Care Providers, Community partners, Family Decision Makers) and encouraging them to become competent in cultural care to foster collaboration. This advocacy work resulted in developing the Collaborative Cultural Competence (C3) in the ACP framework. The hope is that this framework will motivate funders of public health issues to support such community led initiatives.

Essential VI: Interprofessional Collaboration for Improving Patient and Population Health Outcomes. Through interprofessional collaboration, the author improved advance care planning behaviors among

Participants, which is reported to have good health outcomes at the end of life. The author collaborated with the Pastor, the Clerk of "Session," and the congregants at the site. The author also collaborated with community nurses and mental health counselors who were part of the community. The author consulted with content experts and acted as the project leader. The findings of the QI study may be used to influence or change policies that affect ACP behaviors and Advance Directive Completion.

Essential VII: Clinical Prevention and Population Health for Improving the Nation's Health. The eighth Essential places the nursing profession at the core of addressing community, public, and global health issues and problems. The author implemented the quality improvement project with the affected population and evaluated the effectiveness of the interventions. Overall, 47% of participants experienced a change in at least one of the ACP behaviors; appointed an HCP, communicated what was vital to their Health Care Provider, communicated their wishes with family/friends, and or completed the HCP document. Engaging more faith communities will result in good health outcomes for the communities and the Nation. Given that this framework improves readiness to engage in ACP behaviors, it is likely to work with other public health issues such as vaccine hesitancy.

Essential VII: Advance Nursing Practice. The author consulted with the Capstone experts, mentored other healthcare professionals in the community, investigated current health care problems, planned, and executed an intervention to reduce the gap in care, and disseminated knowledge to the community and the nursing profession through manuscript submission. The author held presentations to disseminate results with faculty, peers, and the community to create awareness on evidence-based interventions that can facilitate sustainable outcomes and impact practice. All activities under the first seven Essentials contribute to this requirement.

Implications for Advanced Practice

While the emphasis on ADs in Nursing Education and practice environment is encouraged, more attention needs to be put in the affected population setting to get expected outcomes (improved Readiness to engage in ACP conversations and AD completion). This addresses the DNP's organizational and systems leadership for quality improvement (essential II) and inter-professional collaboration for improving patient and population health outcomes (essential VI).

Although there has been an increasing interest in research in advance care planning and its benefits to patients and the health care system, there are limited investigations per evidence to explore factors outside the clinical settings that account for variations in AD possession among African Americans.

Linking the existing systems to work in synergy benefits the individual and the health care system. Suppose health care workers focus interventions on increasing ADC discussions and AD completion at the bedside. In that case, an opportunity is missed to engage the larger population in the community, especially as African Americans are reportedly seeking care under emergent situations. Health care policy that recognizes the role of faith leaders and community partners in impacting the health of the members of their community widens health systems to meet minority populations. For instance, having grants available to train community leaders in identifying public health issues affecting their communities the most and launching health campaigns to heal health care professionals in those communities.

Conclusion

The purpose of this QI project was to use a multi-modal (live discussions, prints, and educational video) intervention to improve ACP behaviors among African Americans in the community. There was initial confusion on what constituted an Advance Directive and whether individuals could change their minds. Evidence suggested varied factors impact ACP discussions and AD possession. The factors go beyond Health Seeking behaviors, from physical and socio-economic to psycho-spiritual elements. When looking specifically at the African American population, this project's outcomes not only confirm the best evidence-based interventions that could increase AD completion among African Americans. It provides information suggesting the complexity of the issue and calls for additional research in this population to fully understand barriers to the gap in care.

To appropriately understand how African Americans view AD and the barriers to completing an AD, faith leaders and health care professionals in the faith-based community should be considered helpful community partners when planning care for the African American population. The overall effectiveness of the "Honoring Your Choices" QI project may be understated due to the limited time the author had to gather data for activities that may take time, for instance, time to schedule doctor's appointments or to speak with family members. The outcomes of this QI project add to the evidence that, when seeking to increase ACP in the African American patient population, a multi-modal approach is used, and the intervention(s) be community-led.

PART 2:

African American Perspectives on Advance Care Planning Discussions and Advance Directive Completion

African American Perspectives on Advance Care Planning Discussions and Advance Directive Completion

Evidence suggests that African Americans' HSB is responsible for their lack of AD completion. However, there is an insufficient effort by the authors to explain why. Even though an insider and a health care professional, I did not fully understand the magnitude of the problem with low AD completion in the African American community until after implementing the QI project. It became apparent that there was an increased need to reach the African American communities besides the health care professionals who design programs.

This chapter explores possible reasons for the barriers to discussing ACP or completing AD. These behaviors include appointing an HCA, discussing goals of care and treatment with family and health care providers, and completing AD, in a process elaborated in chapter one. The author interviewed a few Americans of African origin about their views on ACP discussions and AD completion. The interviewees were all adults who have had permanent residency and citizenship in America between five and forty years.

The interviewees all have above high school education. Their occupations include nursing, personal care attendant (PCA), security officer, and engineering. The interviewees identified with the following countries of origin: Cameroon, Ghana, Liberia, Sierra Leone, Kenya, South Africa, and Nigeria between January 28, 2022, and March 2, 2022.

The author informed the interviewees of the reason for the conversation to understand their perspective and their community members about ACP and AD completion. They consented to have their names against their shared views, except one which represented their views anonymously. Because these are real people with real stories, the author wanted to give them credit for their stories while protecting the identity of the individuals in their stories. For this reason, the author used only their first names. Note that this activity was not part of the QI project in Part 1. Instead, it was motivated by the "Honoring your Choices" project outcome.

I had told my spouse that I would initiate the AD conversation with the African American community. His response was, "You have the guts not only for choosing that topic but also for choosing this population." And then I asked, how did we get here?

He said it's not something we talk about. Our forefathers informed trusted elders what they wished to happen if they died by word of mouth. It was never what to do *if they become sick*. Partly because we grew up in a health system that lacked preventive care, and the technology was insufficient to prolong life. "Kinsmen" or relatives will come up and decide what was best for the following royalty.

He added that, then, the health care system wasn't sophisticated to worry about its ability to prolong life. As such, the worry was not death (which was natural) but what to do in the event of death. These days, advancements in medical technologies have allowed prolonging lives, and things have changed. Due to the rise of economic values, self-centeredness, and corruption, "the words of the word" must be backed by written documentation of the individual's wishes to avoid conflicts. People will come up and say something contradictory about people's desires. It happens especially in large families. Written documentation is becoming essential to express wishes.

Discussion with Sherley, Nurse (a Liberian American Perspective):

Q. What is your perspective of the ACP conversation and AD completion in the Liberian American community?

A. We don't discuss that! Woe on to you who plan to ask a parent or family member if they have AD. It gets worse if they are wealthy. They will think you are planning to kill them to take their capital. It is a challenging conversation in our community. And I think it's because of lack of education.

We (you and I) are educated and have traveled and got introduced to the way others (like here in America) do things, so we are aware of the benefits. It's not the same for others who are educated in other fields. They have an even stronger opinion than those who are not as educated because we still believe in word of mouth hear-say instead of reading the facts. So, people may be enlightened in general and not informed in ACP.

Thankfully, I worked in health care and was exposed to the ACP process. And am glad for this because I was able to ask my mom if she had a will when she visited me in the States. After encouraging her to write a will and designate who she wished to care for, her health matters if she becomes very sick. She listened. She did not do it then. She returned home, and when on her dying bed, I again asked if she had done it, and she hastily did one. I felt terrible I didn't speak to her sooner before she got sick. Luckily, she could draft a will before she passed because she died. My sibling and I saw uncles we never knew existed. I was glad I had the will in my hand to follow through with her wishes.

In our community, when someone dies, we focus on collecting monies from here and there to pay for the person's funeral home fees. We see the White man, while alive, paying for the funeral home and buying their burial plot. We must contribute money to bury some people. We don't do life insurance and don't plan.

Sherley added; when I did my community project as a student, I decided to pick on a Flu Clinic project to access the large Liberian––American community in the Lowell region. Most of the participants shared they were not taking the flu shot because it made people sick and thought they couldn't get it if they didn't have health insurance. I even attended one of their churches and spoke to the parishioners about the benefits of getting flu shots.

Our culture plays a significant role in that Liberians don't have primary care doctors back at home. Therefore, they cannot afford a primary care visit to hospitals when very sick. I trained mid-wife and worked as a mid-wife for five years in Ghana. Ghana has a better system because they have community and public health nurses in Well Baby Clinics. The latter follows children at birth to five years old in the community to ensure they get all their immunizations. Besides this, people from Liberia and Ghana do not have time for general primary care or dental care.

Again, because they have the cash and care system, not everyone can afford health care. Therefore, traditional medicine, which is less expensive, is often rendered. The influence of tradition is noticeable when individuals prefer to seek the fetish priest than the doctor. For instance, if someone had a boil, they would choose to have a plant leaf squeezed on it than have the doctor drain the boil or abscess. People say that you will likely die if the doctor cuts it open.

Q. Given this cultural background, how do Liberian Americans access to care or complete the AD?

A. Here, if someone is sick and goes to the hospital, the nurse explains what is important and listens. But do they always complete it? NO! I think they don't work because of our mentality toward each other. We often think that someone in the family is jealous of us and wants to kill us. How do you begin to choose someone to act as your HCP if you think they are jealous of you? Trust me, when people realize they can designate an HCP, they will. And once there is conflict, they will change the HCA. Education! Education, education is vital!

Education continues to be the primary vehicle because our people (Liberian Americans), like most Black people, do not trust the "Whiteman" since the time of the Syphilis chaos. Suppose more Black doctors or Black health care professionals take on education. In that case, they will get better outcomes because the

Black patients hear from someone who understands where they are coming from. For instance, I worked in an Emergency Department before. We had a frequent Black patient who was genuinely needy and difficult to care for. She gave a hard time to White nurses, and once on schedule, she was automatically assigned to me. When I spoke with her, I found she did not trust the White nurses because when she said she was in pain, there was that preconceived notion that she was a drug-seeking patient. She felt I wasn't judgmental and treated me differently. Also, my dad, who is still alive, is one of those I need to convince to complete an AD or a will. Whenever I bring up the topic, he will say, "Are you the one who will tell me what to do"?

Last year, my cousin had cancer. When I spoke with her, she hadn't appointed an HCP yet. She had reached out to me to become her HCP. She has an adult daughter and a brother. It wasn't until I took time to find out why any of them had not completed the HCP form with her that I realized it was because the daughter and brother were afraid that it would mean her life would be in their hands. They felt it was burdensome for them. But because I was ready and willing, I became her HCA. I made time and spoke with them, especially as they needed to understand the new drug trials she was exploring at the time. They listened. Individuals are afraid family members will blame them should something go wrong. It is a tough conversation for them to consider.

Suspicion of each other is another barrier! Will completing an HCP mean they have to give access to their bank account information to the HCA? We need more education. People listen, but will they, do it? The good thing is the few who do will make a difference.

Discussion with Lansana, Nurse (a Sierra Leonean Perspective):

Q. What is the state of AD completion among Sierra Leoneans in America?

A. From what I can recall from my great grandfather, grandfather, and father, nothing is down. Culturally and traditionally, the eldest son is the next of kin when the father dies. If a chief, the brother becomes chief. Regardless of the parent's educational status, they rarely wrote anything down. For instance, when my dad passed, my elder brother became the next of kin. He then gave directives on what needed to be done, including the burial. If the next of kin wishes, he could denote the parent's organs. We never have a parent write it down somewhere that "donate my organs. "These days, as the younger generations learn to copy the Western ways of doing things, some people may be writing directives down today.

Q. Have you seen or heard other Sierra Leoneans in your community in Washington DC talk about assigning themselves HCA or other forms of AD?

A. Not really. It is scarce. I have told my spouse to take my remains home if I die. She knows.

Q. Have you also thought of writing the wishes down?

A. (laughter) She knows not to leave my body here, to take me to Sierra Leon and rest me by my dad. It is not written down. Now, you too know, in case she forgets.

Discussion with Evonne, (a Cameroonian American Perspective):

Q. What experiences do you have with ACP or AD or wills?

A. When I was 18 years old, in the village of Ponying Cameroon, my mother was sick on her dying bed and kept sending me. I think she did not want me to see her dying. She first asked that I get some clothes for her; when I returned, she asked me to get her water or something she didn't need at that time. And then, finally, she opened my palm and poured some of the water inside. She said I should take care of my siblings. She wanted me to be her successor, but my younger brother had to because I got married to a foreigner and moved out of the village.

However, my next experience was when one of my uncles who preferred one of his sons, became sick and was hospitalized for some time. The "favorite" son did not show concern for him. He was cared for by his daughter daily in the hospital. He changed his will for whom he wanted to become his heir while at the hospital. My uncle told his best friend that the family should crown his daughter the heir if anything happens. When he finally passed, his friend did not share with the family his will. The family went ahead and made the son the successor. The son died shortly after.

The family made his second son the heir second son became heir, and he too passed. My uncle finally appeared to be his best friend in his dream. He whipped the friend for not informing the family that he had chosen the daughter as his successor. The next day, the best friend ran to some of our family members and announced that uncle told him that the daughter was the successor. He did not inform the family because it was not the norm to have females as successors in our tradition. He had decided to keep this to himself because it was not our tradition to have female heirs.

During this time, the compound in the village was deserted because mysterious things were happening. If one harvested plantains from the yard, their hands became bent or deformed. People avoided coming into the compound for fear of facing the unsettling spirits of uncle. His daughter was the only one who visited the compound, cleaned it, and harvested food from the backyard without issues with the spirits. His dead spirit was at peace with the daughter. The family was relieved and made the daughter his heir. Since then, there has been peace in the compound. The words of those days are more powerful than those of these days; I don't know why.

Interview with Louisa, nurse (Ghanaian Perspective);

Q. What is your experience with ACP and AD completion in your community?

A. We don't talk about it. Death is sacred to us. You are not God to know when someone will plan to plan for it. We don't play God. Every time I teach my patients and need to do ACP with them, I do the teachings alright, though I may not take to the advice I am giving others. If a parent is dying, the children leave the parent to go through the natural process of dying. Suppose one of them was where the HCP is. In that case, they still may not make any significant decisions because they won't want to blame the rest of the family if something goes wrong. Somehow the HCP will be accused to killing the parent.

Take an actual scenario involving a lady I will call Mrs. Smith in her eighties. She was diagnosed with cancer and continued chemotherapy treatments which were not working well for her. I asked one of the children, her HCP, why she continued to let her have the drug. You know what? Though she was the HCP, the brother decided that treatment was continuous.

Another thing, though not scientific, is that there is a fear every time there is death. We (Africans in general) fight till the end because we don't know how to live our lives happily. Every time you see an average to do African, they build a house or do a project. Going to restaurants is even looked at as wasting money that would have been added to a carry out a project. Our lives are often a struggle such that when it gets closer to the end, we hope it is time to begin to enjoy the fruit of our labor. So, we fight and fight till the end. If a child goes to the parent and asks about their wishes, they may call the child "witches" looking forward to their death.

Again, here is this. There was an instance where an elderly mother was diagnosed with cardiac conditions. Her child knew that her time was near due to her advanced age and advanced state of the disease. So, the child had a conversation with the mother about her wishes and whether she should like to be taken back to Ghana, where she will be with many family members and comfort. The mother became upset and invited an interpreter to her doctor visits and let her child accompany her to the clinic. When she finally passed here, it was the child's responsibility and burden to raise the money to send her corpse home, approximately $13,000 for the transportation.

When I started working as a young nurse in a nursing home, it was confusing why patients would choose Do Not Resuscitate (DNR), and Do Not Intubate (DNI), while seeking care. It was because our system did not educate us like that. Although education needs to happen, I am not sure where you begin with this type of education. My community especially needs it. Please find time to speak with people in my community.

Discussion with Calvin, Nurse (a Cameroonian Perspective):

Q. Could you kindly share with me what experiences you have had with ACP discussions and AD completion in your community?

A. For me, it was a surprise when my grandmother, before her passing, would call me, and we would discuss her wishes should she pass away. Because of the structure of our polygamous family, she was motivated to construct her wishes known before she died. And it saved us (family a lot of headaches) though you will always have someone opposes a will in most situations. But once family members see the will with a signature, it is sealed. We still are far behind in planning for care. Culturally, it is a tough sell because people in our community feel that when you put a family member on Hospice, you are killing them. We need to break this cultural barrier to get a common ground in the American health system. The ACP is a timely conversation for our community.

Discussion with Joy, health care worker, (a Nigerian American Perspective):

Q. Do you and members of your community have ACP discussions or complete the HCP?

A. For me, I have completed my HCP, and one of my sons is my HCP. There is increasing development in this area in that individuals are now electing to have wills and life insurance. We don't do much of what I see is common among Cameroonians to take home mortal remains. More people buy life insurance and do not rely on donations to take the mortal remains home. I have even told my family that I would like to be buried in the United States should anything happen to me.

To us (Nigerians), the soul is gone when someone dies. Even my mom (91 years old), appoints one or two of her children as her HCP depending on where she is at the time. I am activated as her HCP if she is with me. If she goes to any other state, that person acts as her HCP.

Anonymous, Nurse (a South African American Perspective)

Q. How do people in your community approach ACP discussions and AD completion?

A. This is one of those topics that people are not comfortable talking about. People assume that once you talk about it, something bad will happen. I am somewhat comfortable talking about it. I have life policies and have planned for the future, but ACP is something I haven't finalized. My husband and I have talked about it.

Anonymous, Sales Associates (a Moroccan American Perspective)

Q. How do you and members of your community feel about ACP discussions?

A. If it is back in Morocco, I will tell you we have a more robust community there than here. Here, it's all about making money, and people don't care about others. For that reason, I am not part of the Moroccan community here. Many Moroccans in the Revere area, and I don't associate with them. The doctors here also are not very flexible. They focus on what is on the paper and sometimes forget about what is in front of them.

Q. Are you saying you feel that the doctor only focuses on the paper regardless of the situation once written?

A. I think the doctors here practice differently.

Q. Are you aware that once a HCP is signed, you can change your mind at any time?

A. Not sure.

Jane, nurse (a Kenyan American Perspective)

Q. What experiences do you have with ACP discussions and AD completion in your community?

A. (laughs) It is a difficult conversation to have. I once worked at a long-term care facility where a resident of African descent was admitted following hospitalization for an acute episode. She was young and, on record, had an HCP. But unfortunately, the HCP was the ex-husband. He did not want anything to do with her anymore, worst still, to make health care decisions on her behalf. It was a sad situation. Updating your HCP is as vital as creating a new HCP people; as time goes by, people change, things change.

Kenyans are beginning to talk about ACP though it's only talking. They don't act on it. So, I talk about it, and I haven't completed mine yet. I even asked my husband his preferences for treatments that prolong life without necessarily improving quality. He said he wants it all for treatment. I asked him whether that means long-term g-tube feedings and tracheostomy. He said, "Yes!" He wants the treatment available to keep him alive. But guess what? If something happens to me before him, he is doomed because I am the only one who knows about this wish and will not write it down.

Someone was on national television speaking to Kenyans about the importance of AD a few days ago. People listen. But they don't act.

Personal Experiences with Advance Directives

I was surprised by how unprepared my family was regarding ACP discussions when our father (Njango) became sick and received medical care in America. Like most African Americans, an educated man himself, it wasn't an easy conversation to have with him. On several days Njango was transferred to the Emergency Medical Department for his heart health issues. A doctor asked me who his HCP was. Although he was mentally alert, the doctors wanted to ensure a completed HCP on file. I felt honored to be part of his care team and consenting on his behalf for treatments as he had many procedures which were invasive.

It was also burdensome in that for every consent given, I feared, "what if something went wrong and he passes because of the procedure? "Yet, it felt better when provided with his disease prognosis, making the procedures lifesaving, thus easier to make. At one time, Django's heart rate was in the thirties instead of being in the range sixty to hundred, and the doctor stated, "He can drop down any time from this hour." Therefore, it made it easier to elect for a pacemaker.

Not so fast! One would think the author acting as the HCP would just consent to a major procedure like that. After working in long-term care facilities, I witnessed many families' dynamics coming into play when patients were at end-of-life. I saw how siblings rival to be part of a parents' care mostly because they wanted to be involved in the decision-making process. However, when an HCP was appointed for a patient, that person became the patient's representative. Because Njango had sons in America, it became imperative that the son gets informed of treatment goals and presumed approval for significant procedures. Despite the understanding that the son cares about his father and trusts the HCP's decisions on behalf of Njango, the plan of care was often shared with the older son per customary ways. And his voice was important in the process. Therefore, the decision wasn't solely the HCA's even when invoked.

When Njango was alert enough in the hospital, I attempted on two occasions to ask what his wishes were on comprehensive terms to initiate the conversation. Instead, he somewhat joked about it and changed the topic. I was scared to proceed with the discussion because he may interpret my inquiry to mean he was dying. We may have lost hope or indicated a lack of compassion. Njango had plans to return to Cameroon in a few weeks. I provided bedside education to my patients about the process and importance of completing AD. This time, it was paralyzing to know the right course of action. Yet, I could not have Njango complete a care directive that met his personal goals in life because I was not a nurse but acting as a child. And then, it became too late to hear from him what he truly wanted "comfort" versus "longevity."

Njango had a massive personality at different levels nationally. Though he had an important role in the politics and economics of Cameroon, he was very humble and charitable. Others had always served him in official settings. However, he served individuals from every level of the socio-economic class, paying more attention to the less privileged. His philanthropic works are discussions for another time.

However, Njango was very anxious when female caregivers were providing care. He had always had a male paid staff to care for his clothes, undergarments, and bedroom. For instance, though with his wife by his side, Njango would prefer to have his son-in-law help with care than his wife.

At first, we (family) laughed about it when he would use his good sense of humor to reject help from female nurses by asking the son-in-law, "What will the pretty nurse do if it stands during care? The Family became concerned and took it seriously when his anxiety increased during care. The female caregivers would describe his agitation as a sign of non-compliance with care. What if there were other important things about how he wanted to receive his care? My mind would question, would he have elected for palliative and hospice care sooner if he understood and had the opportunity to choose? Would Njango have chosen the "Do not

Intubate" (DNI) or "Use long term tracheostomy" if he understood what they meant? All these questions kept playing in my head because the care goals for this "giant" who was now bedridden seemed conflicting with his personality. A personality of one who loved life, never seated, always splitting an orange to share with another person. But one thing was obvious. His family gave him the best care they could, having home care services, his wife, and children at his bedside. The question whether Njango got patient-centered care at end-of-life is one no one has a response to because his care goals were never discussed or written when he was alert enough to do so. This scenario is classic and typical for most Africans. The question becomes, what do we learn from each situation? Does sharing these stories and perspectives mean anything to the reader?

When it was time to pick a Capstone project topic to fulfill a requirement of the Doctorate Degree program, it was clear what I wanted to do. I had so many questions about what made it difficult for African Americans to engage in ACP conversations or complete AD. I was also interested in understanding if the barriers differed for Americans with different geographical regions of origin, thus developing interest to have conversations noted in this section.

Suppose you were a health care professional designing QI projects to increase ACP discussions and AD completion in the African American population. Will you do it differently after understanding the impact of cultural factors?

PART 3

Systems Approach to Increasing Readiness to Engage in Advance Care Planning Discussions and Advance Directive Completion

Systems Approach to Increasing Readiness to Engage in Advance Care Planning Discussions and Advance Directive Completion

The increased legislature and health policies are needed to resolve or close health care access gaps. The recent move in Massachusetts to have Nurse Practitioners practice as independent practitioners is a step forward in recognizing the profession of nursing as a part of the solution to the public health crisis. It becomes vital to support the public health infrastructures and utilize systems thinking approach with interventions. It is also essential to operationalize it to sustain the outcomes in an extended period to realize actual changes that close the gaps.

The American Association of Colleges of Nurses (AACN, 2006) laid principles called "Essentials" of Doctoral Education for advanced nursing practice. The practice focused principles include:

1. Nursing science and theory; scientific underpinnings for practice

2. Systems thinking, health care organizations, and the Advanced Practice Nurse

3. Clinical scholarship and evidence-based practice

4. Information systems/technology and patient care technology for the improvement and transformation of health care

5. Health care policy for advocacy in health care

6. Interprofessional Collaboration for improving patient and population health outcomes

7. Clinical prevention and population health for improving the Nation's health

8. Advanced Nursing Practice

According to the AANC, the DPN graduate is equipped to design, influence, and implement health care policies and advocate for health care policies that addresses issues of social justice and health equity.

Collaborative Cultural Competence (C3) in ACP

When the concept of culture is often used in health care, the connotation of understanding the patient's values and traditional practices comes to play. Cultural competence in this context includes the dual responsibilities of the health professional and patient in understanding each other's culture. Although the burden lies on the professional to be competent clinically, ethically, and culturally, the patient needs to understand traditional practices that may be barriers to their health care system.

The Nursing curriculum should pay attention to and increase the culturally sensitive skills of the novice nurse and nursing students. This would help them understand their cultural practices and biases that may hinder engaging patients in ACP discussions. In addition, health care professionals in the community and primary care clinics could initiate ADC conversations when patients visit for wellness checkups or follow up on chronic issues.

If the opportunity is missed and the patient shows up in an acute care setting, the health professionals have reduced opportunity to explore ACP topic from a proactive perspective. Instead, it became reactive and may be nerve-wracking to the patient when the provider brings up the topic; does it mean I am actively dying? Worst still, presenting to the Emergency Department without an AD while in an unconscious or incapacitated state. Then, it becomes too late for the health professional and the patient to draft a patient-centered care plan.

Madeleine Leininger's (2006) theory of culture care diversity and universality stress the importance of culture in caring. Leininger indicated in her theory that, while it is important for the physiological, psychological, spiritual, and social needs of a patient to identified, it is also important to get the cultural perspective of the patient. To provide holistic care to patients, cultural assessments can tell how much values and beliefs have passed from one generation, down to another which are still impactful to care and outcomes. Culturally competent care means the nurse is responsible for understanding their own cultural values while seeking to understanding those aspects of care that are universal and specific to the patient.

Inspired by Kolcaba's Comfort theory, the author designed the Collaborative Cultural Competence in Advance Care Planning (C3 in ACP) framework. The framework describes the mega health care system and its intervening variables, which work to realize positive HSB in the targeted population. Refer to Chapter 1 for details.

The American health system is superior in technological know-how yet faces challenges in providing equitable care compared with other developed countries. The health systems operate in isolation, and the cost of care or treatment differs for the same ailment in different health systems. Since efforts were made to include social determinants of health into health assessments and billing schemes in the Obama era, the geography of the American health system has changed. Different health systems are seriously considering a call for more population-driven initiatives and a value-based reimbursement model. Covid-19 pandemic precipitated discussions on better furnishing care and getting reimbursed. Providers who hadn't invested in population health and a values-based approach were faced with difficulty meeting their patients' needs, which Telehealth most often dictated.

Although the QI project The Honoring Your Choices Project was implemented in a community setting, the outcomes are gains that can be realized in the acute care and primary care settings at the individual, community, and system levels.

Individually focused, the health professional identifies the physiological needs of patients. Recall that when an individual has a severe or chronic illness that results in frequent hospitalizations, that individual is more likely to be introduced to ACP discussions. In addition, prior studies may have identified specific populations as high risk for particular conditions or poor health outcomes on health measures. The Advanced Practice Nurse's role is to identify the gap in care, possible causes, and barriers and then design interventions to target the identified issue. The focus is to remove the barriers to care and make quality care accessible and equitable.

Lastly, the systems-focus approach doesn't deal with any specific setting (community, acute or primary). It involves the different systems working together on the issues at hand. When the author launched the Honoring Your Choices project, the focus was to find a systems approach to the problem. There was already enough evidence from synthesis on ACP discussions, AD completion, and end-of-life comfort. It was clear that the African Americans' HSB contributed to the low ACP discussions and AD completions. However, there were limited efforts in the research to explore why. Interventions that were mostly designed for the bedside or in acute care settings were continuously used with the hope to increase AD for patients, not necessarily for the African American population.

To understand the barriers to possessing an AD, the author incorporated Kolcaba's Comfort theory concepts, which described the nurse's role in identifying the problem. The theory also describes how the nurse's intervention results to positive HSB and ultimately enhanced comfort.

At the micro-level, the intention of education to both health professionals and the population of interest is to create self-awareness on possible barriers and achieve positive changes in ACP behaviors. At the macro level, bringing the Primary care setting, acute care settings, nursing homes (part of the mega health system) with community partners, legislatures and policymakers will impact the larger national and global strategy. The question is, how do we operate within the current subsystems to maximize health outcomes? Collaboration between and amongst the systems is proven to work well for public and community health issues. See the figure of the suggested Collaborative Cultural Competence (C3) in Advance Care Planning framework below.

Figure 4: Collaborative Cultural Competence (C3) in Advance Care Planning Model

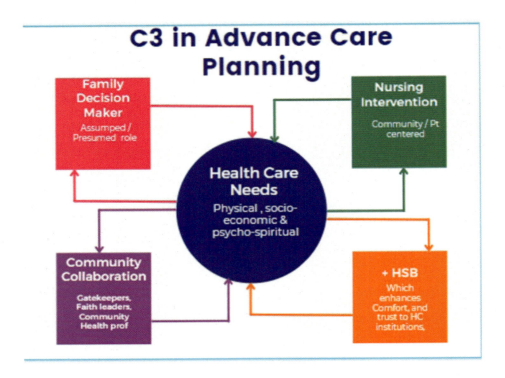

The patient or the community is at the model's center to make it patient-centered. Once the nurse identifies the needs of the patient/population, interventions are designed to meet those needs. In this study, the APN identified the need for ACP in the African American population created the Honoring Your Choices project to increase ACP discussions and AD completion among African Americans. Understanding what common ACP behaviors involve in general and particularly for this population was essential to target the interventions. Suppose participants (the community) became more aware and knowledgeable about ACP and its process, became more ready to engage in the ACP discussions, and complete ADs. In that case, the expected outcome is enhanced comfort at end-of-life. This model is not limited to ACP; it can be used when designing public health interventions in general. And it works for the simple reason that sharing goals and treatment preferences is considered a gift of clarity to the patient health care professionals and the family.

A Gift of Clarity: How?

A Gift of Clarity to the patient/ population

Regardless of the types of wishes, making them known is paramount because even as a member of a population or community, there are variations in values and beliefs. Take for instance: if Pa Tamufor, a patient who is seventy-five years old, feared surgery so intensely that he thought it would kill him or reduce his quality of life, it's all up to him to share what his treatment preferences are to his family and his health provider. By discussing his wishes not to have surgery no matter what, he is sure to die in dignity, only he can define.

However, Abu Makah, who is eighty-five years old and enjoys living, may share with her family that she has cancer and that she wishes to have the best treatments available to prolong her life because she intends to attend her granddaughter's wedding in seven months. Abu Makah has made her treatment goals clear to her family and her care team. The expected outcome of Abu's AD is psychological comfort than physical comfort because it is more important to be present for her granddaughter's wedding. Abu Makah will be at peace knowing her wishes are being honored.

A gift of clarity to the family

Suppose individuals discuss care goals with family members and trusted friends and complete AD. In that case, they are making their wishes known with expectations on things to do should they become unable to make decisions for themselves. For example, it is common to hear of family disputes between each other and between family members and health providers when a patient becomes incapacitated due to a serious illness or an accident. Of course, family members want to give the best care to their loved ones. But their perspective of what quality of care means may be different from the patient's.

Whether based on good intentions or selfish aims, when a patient's goals in care are not known, it's left for the loved ones to advocate for the patient in their own way. The end result is often guilt for the family members regardless of their decision. For instance, Mami Araboh is diagnosed with breast cancer and critically ill without ACP. Her son, the head of household among two other children, automatically is expected to make health care decisions on Mami Araboh's behalf. The doctor advises that a surgery is recommended. The son knows it's the only option to keep the cancer from spreading. Mami gets the surgery done, but cancer has already spread, and she passes on. The presumed HCA feels guilty that maybe the surgery he authorized hastened Mami's death. The siblings blame their HCP for permitting a treatment that allegedly "killed" their mother. If Mami Alaboh had approved invasive treatments for herself with the complete understanding of the implication, she would have given some sense of clarity to her family. If not, the HCP needs to understand what Mami's wishes are by initiating this difficult conversation.

If a family member assigns you to become their HCP, you should be asking "what are your wishes?" What is it you will like me to do, should you become unable to make decisions for yourself? What is important to you? Would you prefer the doctor and the HCP to determine what is best for you at the time? Would you prefer to have any treatment regardless of its invasiveness, or choose not to have long term invasive procedures? And what flexibility do you give your HCP? All, some or none? That is, would you want the HCP to carry out your wishes exactly as shared? Suppose the individual appointing the HCP does not communicate wishes with them. In that case, it is wise for the HCP to bring up the conversation for clarity.

A gift of clarity to the health care professionals

When health care professionals are caring for patients with no ADs on record, the health professionals may be faced with some ethical dilemmas. These includes principles of beneficence (to do good), non-maleficence (not harm), autonomy and justice. The health professional can only provide informed consent (freedom of choice) to the patient is they are mentally sound. Suppose the patient is not physically and mentally sound to give consent. In that case, the HCA will be activated or invoked to represent the patient. Suppose the health professional cannot get consent for treatment simply because the patient had not indicated an HCA. In that case, they are faced with their oath to do the right thing. Keep in mind that because health professionals come from varied cultural and belief systems, what is considered "right thing" may be different for the different health professionals. For example; while one nurse may feel that it is hurtful to administer Cardiopulmonary resuscitation (CPR) to a ninety-five years old bed-bound patient, another nurse may think that it every life is worth saving regardless.

Suppose invasive procedures need to be done on a patient without an HCP. In that case, the health care professional may need time set aside to search for a family member or get a court-appointed guardian to act as an HCP. This takes valuable time from care initiation and puts the health professional in a stressful place. A shared plan of care which is documented gives clear expectations on care goals to the health care providers. The essence of appointing an HCP is portrayed in this actual scenario. An eighty-seven-year-old African American nursing home resident with no appointed HCP on record, continued to receive cancer treatments which are no longer working for him/her. The nursing home managed to get a court appointed guardian to represent the patient because of declined cognitive function. When it was time to discontinue to cancer treatments because the side effects overweighed the benefits, the guardian–attorney could be not reached. The facility is looking to take the case back to court to get another representative. And all the patients can do is wait. Contracted in bed, all I could think about was whether outcomes would have been different if he or she had appointed a family, a friend or a pastor in their community as an HCP to represent them.

Evidence suggested that African Americans have strong community ties. They often see their pastors and members of their churches weekly as opposed to severe months out with their doctors if they do. Their allegiance is to their faith and cultural communities than the health system for many reasons. Thus, it makes sense that if any interventions to increase ACP discussion were being designed; they would be community-led. Faith leaders are the Gatekeepers and should be considered valuable partners in the well-being of African Americans. The C3 in ACP model suggests an integrated system where the Primary Care and Acute Care Centers know who their patients are and the role of religion and faith in their care. Patients without families and trusted friends will likely use their pastors if an option.

Furthermore, a key revealing theme from the project was the idea that, there is a presumed HCP role among African Americans. Family dynamics play a big role in that, it is assumed the head of the family, or the household is in charge of making key decisions for family members, including health care decisions. This means, if the head of household (HOH) doesn't complete an ACP, it is probable that the children or spouse are not thinking of it or not culturally correct to do so. The head of the household is often a male, a fatherly figure, or the oldest son. This may be different when the mother is the one who works in the health care field and understands the process of completing ADs than the male head of household. Either way, the input of the head of household or Family Decision Maker is vital in the process.

Applicability of the Public Health Intervention, or The Intervention Wheels

The Public Health Intervention Wheel, also known as the Minnesota Model, describes the use of public health interventions at different levels of the practice (Wisconsin Department of Health Services, 2022). The Intervention Wheels are often used for disease surveillance and prevention of the spread of infectious diseases. The Wheel is useful and applicable when seeking interventions to reduce the care gaps or tackling public health issues in generals. For example, it is essential to understand where individuals are regarding ACP and finding a middle ground to break barriers. This "surveillance" work is only successful if outreach is done into those affected communities, community-focused, and community-led interventions, and collaboration with subsystems occurs.

The public health intervention wheel is instrumental in applying interventions at various practice levels. Like most public health issues, the Wheel continue to be a vital tool in addressing advance care planning deficit among African Americans. Its applicability includes interventions that are individual, or family focused, community focused, and systems focused. The Planning stage is involved with surveillance (Wisconsin Department of Health Services, 2022). In this case, research local, state, and national prevalence of the issue with ACP. Secondly, investigate the occurrence of the issue and lastly outreach to the affected community. In the implementation phase, screening or assessing understanding of the bottom line, providing health education to the targeted population, refer as needed and lastly, enforce on policies.

Nurse scholars, faculty, and clinicians should collaborate toward an improved and interconnected health system. Transformational leaders who can juggle management and quality in care outcomes are important to close care gaps between patient populations.

The role of the bedside nurse is critical as issues are identified at the bedside. The role of Advance Practice Nurses (APN) in practice settings is crucial at bringing best-evidenced interventions to reduce or close the care gap. The success of a transformational leader lies in their ability to manage the practice systems such that the care rendered is safe, timely, effective, efficient, and patient-centered. In addition, the leader must consider ways to sustain the gains long enough to close the gap via the use of practice conceptual models like the Plan Do Study Act (PDSA).

Conclusion

The author explored (i) the perspectives of health professionals on ACP through literature synthesis, (ii) explored some of the perspectives of Americans of African descent, and (iii) drew from her professional and personal experiences as an attempt to initiate ACP discussions and increase AD completion in the community. However, the author is not suggesting this book as a solution to the public health issue. Instead, this is an initial response to researchers that there is potential for sustained outcomes if barriers to ACP discussion and AD completion are better understood. Once the complexity of the issue of ACP with African Americans is understood, it gives opportunity to advocate for policies that support the structures involved. Supporting local public health initiatives in the communities with training and funding opportunities will improve the collaborative works with health care professionals in the various settings, community members, and partners. Having the opportunity to initiate this conversation is a step in that direction.

The DPN graduate is equipped to design, influence, and implement health care policies and advocate for health care policies that addresses issues of social justice and health equity.

REFERENCES

American Association of Colleges of Nursing (2006). The essentials of doctoral education for advanced nursing practice. Retrieved from Https://www.aacnnursing.org/Portals/42/Publications/DNPEssentials.pdf

Arruda, L. M., Abreu, K. P., Santana, L. B., & Sales, M. B. (2019). Variables that influence the medical decision regarding advance directives and their impact on end-of-life care. *Einstein Journal.* doi:10.31744/Einstein journal/2020RW4852.

Bernacki, R. E., & Block, S. D. (2014). Communication about serious illness care goals: A review and synthesis of best practices. *Journal of American Medical Association. 174 (12),* 1994-2003.

Carson, R.C. & Bernacki, R. (2017). Is the end in sight for the "Don't ask don't tell" approach to advance care planning? *Clinical Journal of the American Society of Nephrology, 12*(1), 380-381. doi:10.2215/CJN.00980117.

Cornally, N., McGlade, C., Weathers, E., Daly, E., Fitzgerald, C., O'Caoimh, R., Coffey, A., & Molloy, W. (2015). Evaluating the systemic implementation of the 'Let Me Decide' advance care planning programme in long-term care through focus groups: Staff perspective. *National Library of Medicine*, doi:10.1186/s12904-015-0051-x.

Davis, C. P. (2021). Medical definition of advance directives. MedicineNet. Retrieved from Https://www.medicincenet.com/advance_directives/definition.htm

Durbin, C. R., Fish, A. F., Bachman, J. A., Smith, K. V. (2010). Systemic review of educational interventions for improving advance directive completion. *Journal of Nursing Scholarship, 42*(3), 234-241. doi:10.1111/j.1547-5069.2010.01357.x.

Fried, T. R., Redding, C., Robbins, M., Paiva, A., O'Leary, J. R. and Iannone, L. (2010). Stages of change for the component behaviors of advance care planning. *Journal of American Geriatric Society, 58*(12), 2329-2336. doi:10.1111/j.1532-5415.2010.03184.x.

Garrido, M. M., Balboni, T. A., Maciejewski, P. K., Boa, Y., & Prigerson, H. G. (2014). Quality of life and cost of care at the end of life: The role of advance directives. *Journal of Pain Symptom Management, 49*(5), 828-835. doi:10.1016/j.painsymman.2014.09.015.

Garritano, N.F., Glazer, G., & Willmarth-Stec, M., 2016. *The Journal for Nurse Practitioners, 12*(4), 143-150

Herdeman, R. R., & Karbeath, J. (2020). Examining racism in health services research: A disciplinary self-critique. *Health Services Research, 55*(2), 777-780. doi:10.1111/1475-6773-13558.

Huang, I. A., Neuhaus, J. M., & Chiong, W. (2016). Racial and ethnic differences in advanced directive possession: Role of demographic factors, religion affiliation, and personal health values in a national survey of older adults. *Journal of Palliative Medicine, 19*(2), 149-156. doi:10.1089/jpm.2015.0326.

Indeed Editorial Team. (2021). Prospective study vs. retrospective study: What are the differences? *Indeed*, Prospective Study vs. Retrospective Study: What Are the Differences? | Indeed.com.

Johnson, K.S., Elbert-Avila, K. I., & Tulsky, J. A. (2005). The influence of spiritual beliefs and practices on the treatment preferences of African Americans: A review of the literature. Journal of American Geriatrics Society, *53*(4). doi:10.1111/j.1532-5415.2005.53224.x.

Klingler, C., Schmitten, J., & Marckmann, G. (2016). Does facilitated advance care planning reduce the cost of care near the end of life? Systemic review and ethical considerations. *Palliative Medicine, 30*(5), 423-433. doi:10.1177/0269216315601346.

Koss, C. S. ,& Baker, T. A. (2017). A question of trust: Does mistrust or perceived discrimination account for race disparities in advance directive completion? *The Gerontological Society of America, 00(00),*1-10. doi:10:1093/geroni/igx017.

Koss, C. S., & Baker, T. A. (2017). Where there's a will: The link between estate planning and disparities in advance care planning by white and black older adults. *SAGE Journals*, *40*(3), 281-302. doi:10.1177/0164027517697116.

Kolcaba, K. (2001). Evolution of the mid-range theory of comfort for outcomes research. *Nursing Outlook*, *49*(2), 86-92. Doi:10.1067/mno.2001.110268.

Kwak, J., & Haley W. E. (2005). Current research findings on end-of-life decision making among racially or ethnically diverse groups. *The Gerontological Society of America*, *45(5)*, 634-6641.

Lakin, J. R., Koritsantszky, L. A., Cunningham, R., Maloney, F. L., Neal, B. J., Paladino, J., Palmor, M. C., Vogeli, C., Ferris, T. G., Block, S. D., Gawande, A. A., & Bernacki, R. E. (2017). A Systematic intervention to improve serious illness communication in primary care. *Health Affairs. 36*(7). doi:10.1377/hlthaff.2017.0219.

Laury, E. R., Greenle, M. M., & G., Meghani, S. (2019). Advance Care Planning Outcomes in African Americans: An empirical look at the trust variable. *Journal of Palliative Medicine*, *22*(4), 442-451. doi:10.1089/jpm.2018.0312.

Leininger, M. (2006). Nursing theorist. *Nursing Theory*. Retrieved from https://nursing-theory.org/nursing-theroies/Madeleine-Leninger.php.

Oskousi, T., Pandya, R., Weiner, D. E., Wong, J. B., Koch-Weser, S., & Ladin, K. (2020). Advance Care planning among older Adults with Advanced non-dialysis dependent CKD and their care partners: perceptions versus reality? *Kidney Medicine, 2*(2), 116-124. doi:10.1016/j.xkme.2019.11.002.

Pollock, K., & Wilson, E. (2015). Care and communication between health professionals and patients affected by severe or chronic illness in community care settings: A qualitative study of care at the end of life. *Health Services and Delivery Research*, *3*(31). Retrieved from Https://www.ncbi.nlm.nih.gov/books/NBK305818/.

Wisconsin Department of Health Services (2022). Public Health Nursing: The Public Health Intervention Wheel. Retrieved from https://www.dhs.wisconsin.gov/phnc/interevntionwheel.htm.

Tah, A. Villeroy (2021) Educational video https://www.canva.com/design/DAEnxNbvceY/C_tU0sn_MnBnbG8kcFwjaQ/watch?utm_content=DAEnxNbvceY&utm_campaign=designshare&utm_medium=link&utm_source=publishsharelink

Vyas, D. A., Eisenstien, L. G., & Jones, D. S. (2020). Hidden in plain sight – Reconsidering the use of race correction in clinical algorithms. *The New England Journal of Medicine*, 874-882. Retrieved from Https://www.nejm.org.

Wickstrom, G., & Bendix T., 2000. The "Hawthorne effect" - What did the original Hawthorne studies actually show? *Scandinavian Journal of Work, Environment and Health*, *26*(4), 363-367.

Yildiz, E. (2019). Ethics in nursing: A systemic review of the framework of evidence perspective. *National Library of Medicine*. Retrieved from https://pubmed.ncbi.nlm.nih.gov/29166840. Doi:10.1177/0969733017734412

APPENDICES

Appendix A: Agreement Letter from Project Site

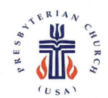

Hartford Street Presbyterian Church

99 HARTFORD STREET
NATICK, MASSACHUSETTS 01760

PHONE: (508) 653-4839
FAX: (508) 653-0762
email: natickpres@aol.com
www.natickpres.org

July 28, 2021

Teresa Kuta Reske, DNP, MPA , RN
Associate Dean of Graduate Studies
Director of the Doctor of Nursing Practice Program
Elms College School of Nursing
291 Springfield Street
Chicopee, MA 01013

Dear Dean Reske,

The Session of Hartford Street Presbyterian Church looks forward to working with Villeroy Tah on her Advance Care Planning quality improvement project, "Honoring Your Wishes." Our understanding is she will do her work in the fall of 2021. This should be a good time at the church, because we should be meeting in person again.

Ms. Tah will be announcing her project in our church newsletter in August. She will also be speaking to the congregation about her project. A tentative plan will be to conduct an information session after church in September, including a brief survey of congregants and the distribution of proxy forms. A second session will be conducted with two to three weeks of the initial one.

Our understanding is that Ms. Tah will also engage in follow-up discussions and distribute materials, such as an educational video, for those who express interest in the program.

We welcome the opportunity to have her conduct part of her project with our church.

Sincerely,

Michael F. Fitzgerald
Clerk of Session
Hartford Street Presbyterian Church
99 Hartford Street
Natick, MA. 01760

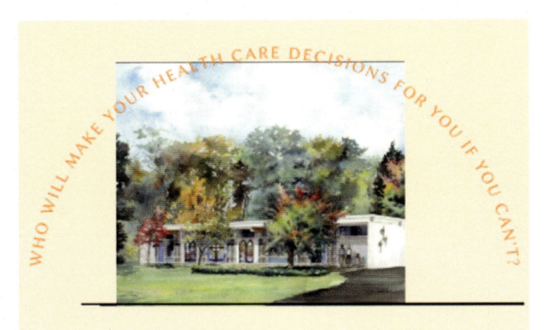

WHO WILL MAKE YOUR HEALTH CARE DECISIONS FOR YOU IF YOU CAN'T?

HONORING YOUR CHOICES

JOIN US AFTER WORSHIP TO LEARN ABOUT ADVANCE CARE PLANNING TO ENSURE YOUR CHOICES ARE HONORED. MAKE THIS A GIFT TO YOURSELF.

Sunday, October 17, 2021
&
Sunday, October 31, 2021
At 11:30 AM (After Service)

Hartford Street Presbyterian Church, 99 Hartford Street, Natick MA 01760

Contact: Villeroy Tah, MSN, RN. Cell: 774 460 1822
Email: tahv@student.elms.edu
Doctor in Nursing Practice (DNP) Capstone Project.
IRB Approval #121020211

Hartford Street Presbyterian Church, Natick MA.

Recruitment Statement for Participation in the Project.

Villeroy Tah, MSN, RN, is inviting you to participate in this quality improvement project.

The title of this project is Honoring Your Choices. The purpose of this project is to improve participants' knowledge of Advance Care Planning (ACP) and readiness to appoint a health care agent, complete a health care proxy document and communicate decisions and choices to their family and doctors. When individuals plan for their care, their choices or preferences for medical treatments will be honored even when they cannot communicate due to serious illness. As a result, their family and doctors will be less confused about treatment preferences, and the cost of their care may be lower.

Your participation in this project will involve:
1. Completing a pre-discussion survey
2. Watching a brief video on how to appoint a health care proxy
3. Sharing your thoughts about advance care planning during discussion sessions
4. Reading a flyer on steps to choose a decision-maker
5. Completing the Massachusetts Health Care Proxy document if desired
6. Completing a post-discussion survey.

Adult congregants at 18 years and older can participate in this project. Participants should be able to speak and understand the English language and be willing to participate in a discussion session on a Sunday after service.

The risks to you as a participant are minimal. Advance care planning discussions may be uncomfortable for some individuals. A national mental health hotline which is available 24 hours a day, seven days a week will be provided should you need to speak with a mental health specialist. In addition, the DNP student (Villeroy Tah) will be available by phone and email to respond to any questions or concerns you may have.

The result of this study may be published in scientific research journals or presented at professional conferences. However, your name and identity will not be revealed, and your record will remain anonymous. Furthermore, your names will not be written or associated with any of the survey responses. Finally, the data collected will be accessible only to the DNP Student and will be stored in a locked cabinet in a locked room.

Participation in this study may benefit you directly by helping you possess the knowledge of ACP and completion of health care proxy. Furthermore, your participation may benefit others indirectly. The data collected will contribute to the analysis of evidence-based practices that improve end of life care of patients in the community setting. Also, your congregation may become equipped and willing to attract and support others in the community with ACP.

You can choose not to participate. If you decide not to participate, there will not be a penalty to you or loss of any benefits to which you are otherwise entitled. You may withdraw from this project at any time.

If you have questions about this study, you can contact Villeroy Tah at 774 460 1822.

Report complaints or grievances regarding this study to the College IRB at irb@elms.edu, and Dr. Teresa Reske, DNP, MPA, RN, Interim Dean, School of Nursing at 413 265 2409.

IRB approval #:121020211

Elms College Doctor of Nursing Practice Program Request for Appointment of DNP Capstone Project Team Member

Elms College DNP Student: *Villeroy Tah, MSN, RN*

DNP Project Title: *Honoring Your Choices*

Date of Submission to the DNP office: *8/21/21*

The DNP Capstone Project Team member(s) was contacted, and their signature indicates a willingness to serve on my DNP Capstone Project Team as follows.

- DNP Capstone Project Chair – The project "Chairperson" is an approved Elms College nursing faculty member who is selected and assigned to the student by the Director of the DNP Program.
- Team Member - The Team Member is a stakeholder in the student's project, an advanced practice nurse/nurse practitioner, provider, or leader who has clinical practice content expertise in the student's area of interest and in particular, the student's DNP Capstone Project focus and population of interest.
- Additional team members – Additional Team members are optional and may be content experts, project reader, or a facilitator at the project site to assist the student in their DNP Capstone Project implementation.

By signing this form, the DNP Capstone Project team member verifies that NO CONFLICT OF INTEREST EXISTS in working with the DNP student nor any investment in their project for personal gains.

1. Chairperson of the DNP Capstone Project Team Approval.
Name: **Dr. Teresa Reske**

_____
Signature   Date

2. DNP Capstone Project Team Member (resume attached).
Name: **Maurine Kisob, BSN, RN**

_____
Signature   Date

Additional Project Team Members (OPTIONAL)

3. Project Team Member. [Print Name, identify the team members, their credentials, role in projects such as (content expert, reader,) organization/facility.]
Team Member's Role: Project Facilitator
Name: **Micheal Fitzgerald, Clark of HSPC Ruling Body (also known as Session).**

_____

Signature   Date

4. Project Team Member. [Print Name, identify the team members, their credentials, role in project such as (content expert, reader,) organization/facility.]

Team Member's name / Role: Maurine Kisob, RN (Health Care Proxy Champion - HCPC). Ms. Maurine is a nurse and a nursing teacher for the novice health care worker who is an active leader in the African American Christian Community in the area.

The HCPC will be available on both discussion sessions to assist Congregants who may need help with completing the HCP document. The HCPC will also assist in sharing paper copies of pre-discussion surveys, HCP brochure, and post discussion surveys to participants to ensure time is maximized. The HCPC should be comfortable with answering questions related to the completion of HCPs.

Team Member's name / Role: Michael Fitzgerald, Clark of Session (Project Facilitator).
 Mr. Fitzgerald is an Editor for the Massachusetts Public Health Organization by profession. Other Facilitator: Rev. Kathie Cole (Pastor of Hartford Street Presbyterian Church).

The Project Facilitator will collaborate with the DNP student at each step of the implementation phase to ensure a smooth medium of communication between the DNP student body of the church (also known as Session) and the rest of the Congregation. The Project Facilitator will assist in making the provided documents, recruitment statement, and educational video are transmitted electronically to the Congregants by group email, on the church website, Newsletter and on the Church Projector screen during announcement time at church service on three Sundays before the start of the project. The Project Facilitator will become a resource person for the Congregation to sustain the project's gains to members and to the Congregation.

Signature Date Approval granted.

Approval: _____
Teresa Kuta Reske DNP, MBA, RN   Date

Pre-discussion survey.   IRB approval #: 121020211

Honoring Your Choices- Project

Honoring Your Choices project at Hartford Street Presbyterian Church, Natick, MA in Fall 2021.

Pre-Discussion Survey:

A Health Care Agent (HCA) can be a trusted family member or friend you may assign to make health care decisions on your behalf should you become unable to make those decisions for yourself. A Health Care Agent is sometimes called a Health Care Proxy (HCP).

When you complete documents that direct doctors on your treatment preferences or which names a family member as your Health Care Agent, you are planning in advance for your care. Advance Care Planning (ACP) can be in the form of a Living Will, Health Care Proxy, Advance Directives, or Durable Power of Attorney for Health Care.

This project focuses on conversations about appointing a Health Care Agent, informing them and your doctors about your choices and decisions, and completing a Health Care Proxy form. The goal is to improve the quality of care you get, especially at the end of life, and of course, honoring your choices.

Before we begin these conversations, please take a few minutes to complete the Pre-Discussion Survey (Questions 1 through 17).

Thank you.

Contact: Villeroy Tah, RN. Cell: 774 460 1822. Email: tahv@student.elms.edu

This survey was modified from the Readiness Scale developed by Fried, T.R., Redding, C., Robbins, M., Paiva, A., O'Leary, J.R., & Iannone, L. (2010).

1

1. Have you appointed a family member or friend who can make decisions on your behalf in the event you are unable to make your own decision because of a serious illness?

- Yes, I have
- No, I haven't
- No, I am uncomfortable to think about it
- I don't need too

2. If you have already talked to family members or friends about your health care decisions, how long ago did this happen?

- Within the past 6 months
- More than 6 months ago
- Not applicable

3. Which of the following types of Advance Care Planning have you completed?

- A Living Will
- Durable Power of Attorney for Healthcare
- Health Care Proxy
- Other (please name it here) _____
- I don't need advance care planning

4. Looking at your answer to Question 3, how long ago did you complete this type of Advance Care Planning?

- Within the past 6 months
- More than 6 months ago
- I am uncomfortable thinking about advance care planning
- I don't need advance care planning

5. Have you talked to your family or friends about medical treatments that prolong life, such as being placed on machines that help you breathe?

- Yes, I have
- No, I haven't
- No, I am uncomfortable thinking about it

6. If you have already talked to family or friends about treatments that prolong life, when did you do this?
- Within the past 6 months
- More <u>than 6</u> months ago
- Not Applicable (N/A)

7. Have you talked to your doctor about what is important to you?
- Yes, I have
- No, I have not
- No, I am uncomfortable talking about this

8. If you have talked to your doctor about what is important to you, when did you do this?

- Within the past 6 months
- More than 6 months ago
- Not applicable

From Question 9 to 14, please select the response that best represents your thoughts:

9. I have the right to refuse medical treatment, even if that treatment might keep me alive longer.
- Agree
- Disagree

10. A Health Care Agent (HCA) is someone who would make medical decisions on my behalf if I were not able to make decisions for myself.
- Agree
- Disagree

11. Once I sign a Health Care Proxy form, I cannot change my mind about how I would want to be treated.
- Agree
- Disagree

3

12. Where is it important to keep a copy of my health care proxy? Choose all that apply.

- At home
- With my doctor
- With a trusted Family member or friend
- All Above

13. A Health Care Proxy is legal if only drawn up by a lawyer.

- Agree
- Disagree

14. If I talk with my doctor about my health care choices and decisions, I don't need to talk to family members too.

- Agree
- Disagree

15. How do you identify yourself?

- Black
- White
- Asian
- Hispanic/Latinx
- Native American
- Pacific Islander
- Other _____

16. How old are you?

- 18 - 28 years
- 29 - 38 years
- 39 - 48 years
- 49 - 58 years
- 59 - 68 years
- 69 - 78 years
- 79 - 88 years
- 89 and over

4

Open link below.

https://www.canva.com/design/DAEnxNbvceY/C_tU0sn_MnBnbG8kcFwjaQ/watch?utm_content=-DAEnxNbvceY&utm_campaign=designshare&utm_medium=link&utm_source=publishsharelink

Fun Facts Shared during discussion.

Discussions: Did You Know that...

*40 % of Older Americans are unable to make their own decisions at end of life?

*2 out of 3 Americans do not have an Advance Directive.

*Black Americans are less likely to possess an Advance Directive (24%) than Hispanics (29%) and Whites (40%).

*Your care may be delayed if health care professionals are unsure about your wishes

*Your family may become stressed to have to make decisions on your behalf if you didn't share your wishes with them?

*Family disputes increase in cases when an individual does not have an advance directive?

*Doctors take your wishes seriously when planning for your care?

*Act Now!! Give yourself and your family a Gift of CLARITY on your wishes, and your Wishes will be Honored.

Need Help Completing the Form?

Ask one of the Collaborators for directions

Congratulations in taking the first Steps in planning for your care when you become unable to make decisions for yourself.

Appendix G: Prepare for Your Care brochure (visit website for details).

PREPARE (prepareforyourcare.org)

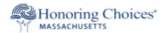 **Honoring Choices®**
MASSACHUSETTS

Massachusetts Health Care Proxy Instructions and Document

Instructions: Every competent adult, 18 years old and older, has the right to appoint a Health Care Agent in a Health Care Proxy. To create your Health Care Proxy, print this two page form and place the instructions page and the blank document in front of you. Follow the step-by-step instructions and sign and date the Health Care Proxy in front of two witnesses, who sign and date the document after you.

1. Your Name and Address *(Required)*
Print your full name in the blank space. Print your address.

2. My Health Care Agent is: *(Required)*
Print the name, address and phone numbers of your Health Care Agent.
- Choose a person you trust to make health care decisions for you based on your choices, values and beliefs, if you cannot make or communicate decisions yourself;
- Your Health Care Agent and Alternate Agent cannot be a person who is an operator, administrator or employee in the facility where you are a patient or resident or have applied for admission, unless they are related to you by blood, marriage or adoption.

3. My Alternate Health Care Agent *(Not required, but helpful to have an Alternate Agent)*
If possible, appoint a person you trust as a back-up or Alternate Agent, who can step-in to make health care decisions if your Health Care Agent is not available, not willing or not competent to serve, or is not expected to make a timely decision. Print the name, address and phone numbers.

4. My Health Care Agent's Authority *(Required)*
Here's where you give your Agent either the broadest possible decision-making authority to make "any and all" decisions including life sustaining treatments, or limit his/her authority:
- If you want to give "any and all" decision-making authority, just leave this area blank.
- If you do not want to give "any and all" decision-making authority, describe the way in which you want to limit your Agent's authority and write it down in the space provided.

5. Signature and Date *(Required)*
Do NOT sign ahead. Sign your full name & date in front of two adult witnesses who sign after you.
- You can have someone sign your name at your direction in front of two witnesses.

6. Witness Statement and Signature *(Required)*
Any competent adult can be a witness except your Health Care Agent and Alternate Agent.
- Two adults must be present as witnesses when this document is signed. They watch as you sign the document, or as another person signs at your direction, and sign after you to state that you are at least 18 years old, of sound mind, and under no constraint or undue influence.
- Have Witness One sign, then print his or her name and the date;
- Then have Witness Two sign and print his or her name and the date.

7. Health Care Agent Statement *(Optional)*
This section is not required, but it can help your doctors and family know the Agents you appointed have accepted the position. Your Agent(s) signs and prints the date in the spaces provided.

Important: Keep your original Health Care Proxy. Make a copy and give it to your Health Care Agent. Give a copy to your doctors and care providers to scan in your medical record so they know how to contact your Agent if you are ill or injured and unable to speak for yourself.

Massachusetts Health Care Proxy

1. I, _____ Address: _____ ,
appoint the following person to be my Health Care Agent with the authority to make health care decisions on my behalf. This authority becomes effective if my attending physician determines in writing that I lack the capacity to make or communicate health care decisions myself, according to Chapter 201D of the General Laws of Massachusetts.

2. My Health Care Agent is:

Name: _____ Address: _____

Phone(s): _____; _____; _____

3. My Alternate Health Care Agent

If my Agent is not available, willing or competent, or not expected to make a timely decision, I appoint:

Name: _____ Address: _____

Phone(s): _____; _____; _____

4. My Health Care Agent's Authority

I give my Health Care Agent the same authority I have to make any and all health care decisions

including life-sustaining treatment decisions, except (list limits to authority or give instructions, if any):

_____

_____

I authorize my Health Care Agent to make health care decisions based on his or her assessment of my choices, values and beliefs if known, and in my best interest if not known. I give my Health Care Agent the same rights I have to the use and disclosure of my health information and medical records as governed by the Health Insurance Portability and Accountability Act of 1996 (HIPAA), 42 U.S.C. 1320d. Photocopies of this Health Care Proxy have the same force and effect as the original.

5. Signature and Date. I sign my name and date this Health Care Proxy in the presence of two witnesses.

SIGNED _____ **DATE** _____

6. Witness Statement and Signature

We, the undersigned, have witnessed the signing of this document by or at the direction of the signatory above and state the signatory appears to be at least 18 years old, of sound mind and under no constraint or undue influence. Neither of us is the health care agent or alternate agent.

Witness One
Signed: _____

Print Name: _____

Date: _____

Witness Two
Signed: _____

Print Name: _____

Date: _____

7. Health Care Agent Statement (Optional):

We have read this document carefully and accept the appointment.

Health Care Agent _____ Date _____

Alternate Health Care Agent _____ Date _____

This Massachusetts Health Care Proxy was prepared by Honoring Choices Massachusetts, Inc.

Appendix I: Advance Directive Notification Card

Advance Directive Notification Card	Advance Directive Notification Card

My Name is: _____
I have the following **Advance Directives**:
    o   Health Care Agent
    o   Living Will
    o   Durable Power of Attorney for Health Care
    o   Advance Directives for Health Care
    o   Other_____
To locate copies of my Advance Directive, contact:
   Name: _____
   Phone #s: _____
Medical Facility or Doctor with copy of my Advance Directive: _____
	I have a Health Care Agent:
	    o **YES**
	        Name: _____
	        Phone #s_____
	
	    o **NO**
	        If I am in an emergency, please contact:
	        Name_____
	        Phone #s_____
	
	Date of notification card completion: _____
	Honoring Your Choices Program
	#121020211

Honoring Your Choices- Project

Honoring Your Choices project at Hartford Street Presbyterian Church, Natick, MA in Fall 2021.

Post-Discussion Survey:

A Health Care Agent (HCA) can be a trusted family member or friend you may assign to make health care decisions on your behalf should you become unable to make those decisions for yourself. A Health Care Agent is sometimes called a Health Care Proxy (HCP).

When you complete documents that direct doctors on your treatment preferences or which names a family member as your Health Care Agent, you are planning in advance for your care. Advance Care Planning (ACP) can be in the form of a Living Will, Health Care Proxy, Advance Directives, or Durable Power of Attorney for Health Care.

This project focuses on conversations about appointing a Health Care Agent, informing them and your doctors about your choices and decisions, and completing a Health Care Proxy form. The goal is to improve the quality of care you get, especially at the end of life, and of course, honoring your choices.

Before we end these conversations, please take a few minutes to complete the Post-Discussion Survey (Questions 1 through 15).

Thank you.

Contact: Villeroy Tah, RN. Cell: 774 460 1822. Email: tahv@student.elms.edu

This survey was modified from the Readiness Scale developed by Fried, T.R., Redding, C., Robbins, M., Paiva, A., O'Leary, J.R., & Iannone, L. (2010).

1

Honoring Your Choices project at Hartford Street Presbyterian Church, Natick, MA in Fall 2021.

Post-Discussion Survey:

You should only complete this section after discussions. Thank you.

1. Have you appointed a family member or friend who can make decisions on your behalf in the event you are unable to make your own decision because of a serious illness?

- Yes, I have
- No, I haven't
- No, I am uncomfortable to think about it
- I don't need too

2. If you have already talked to family members or friends about your health care decisions, how long ago did this happen?

- Within the past 6 months
- More than 6 months ago
- Not applicable

3. Which of the following types of Advance Care Planning have you completed?

- A Living Will
- Durable Power of Attorney for Healthcare
- Health Care Proxy
- Other (please name it here) _____
- I don't need advance care planning

4. Looking at your answer to Question 3, how long ago did you complete this type of Advance Care Planning?

- Within the past 6 months
- More than 6 months ago

- I am uncomfortable thinking about advance care planning
- I don't need advance care planning

5. Have you talked to your family or friends about medical treatments that prolong life, such as being placed on machines that help you breathe?
- Yes, I have
- No, I haven't
- No, I am uncomfortable thinking about it

6. If you have already talked to family or friends about treatments that prolong life, when did you do this?
- Within the past 6 months
- More than 6 months ago
- Not Applicable (N/A)

7. Have you talked to your doctor about what is important to you?
- Yes, I have
- No, I have not
- No, I am uncomfortable talking about this

8. If you have talked to your doctor about what is important to you, when did you do this?

- Within the past 6 months
- More than 6 months ago
- Not applicable

From Question 9 to 14, please select the response that best represents your thoughts:

9. I have the right to refuse medical treatment, even if that treatment might keep me alive longer.
- Agree
- Disagree

3

10. A Health Care Agent (HCA) is someone who would make medical decisions on my behalf if I were not able to make decisions for myself.

- Agree
- Disagree

11. Once I sign a Health Care Proxy form, I cannot change my mind about how I would want to be treated.

- Agree
- Disagree

12. Where is it important to keep a copy of my health care proxy? Choose all that apply.

- At home
- With my doctor
- With a trusted Family member or friend
- All Above

13. A Health Care Proxy is legal if only drawn up by a lawyer.

- Agree
- Disagree

14. If I talk with my doctor about my health care choices and decisions, I don't need to talk to family members too.

- Agree
- Disagree

15. Select one of the following responses as applicable to you:

- I completed a Health Care Proxy document today
- I plan to complete a Health Care Proxy form within the next 3 months
- I plan to complete a Health Care Proxy within the next 6 months
- I don't plan to complete a Health Care Proxy at all

……….The End…….

This survey was modified from the Readiness Scale developed by Fried, T.R., Redding, C., Robbins, M., Paiva, A., O'Leary, J.R., & Iannone, L. (2010).
Contact: Villeroy Tah, RN. Cell: 774 460 1822. Email: tahv@student.elms.edu

4

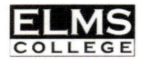

October 12, 2021

Dear Ms. Tah,

Thank you for submitting the IRB documentation for your project entitled "Honoring Your Wishes". Your project has been approved by the Elms College IRB and you may now proceed with data collection.

As principle investigator, it is your responsibility to conduct this study as it was approved by the IRB.

If you plan any changes or modifications to protocol, please submit an "IRB Change of Protocol" form which can be found at the Elms IRB website prior to implementation.

Please note that all further communication regarding this survey should include the **approval #121020211**. Please include this approval number on all of your study documents before commencing data collection.

Upon completion of your data collection, please complete the "IRB Research Closure Form", which can be found on the Elms IRB website.

We wish you success with your project! If you have any questions about this process or need further assistance from the IRB, please contact IRB Chair Dr. Cynthia L. Dakin, RN at dakinc@elms.edu and 413-265-2455.

Sincerely,

Cynthia S Dakin, RN, PhD

Cynthia L. Dakin, RN, PhD
Chair, Elms College Institutional Review Board
Elms College
291 Springfield St.
Chicopee, MA 01013

191 Springfield Street
Chicopee, MA 01013-2839
413-594-2761
www.elms.edu

Villeroy Tah, MSN, RN

Approval #121020211

December 24, 2022

Project Title: Honoring Your Choices

Site: HSPC Natick

Dear HSPC Natick,

C/O Mr. Fitzgerald,

I wish to thank you and the Session of Hartford Street Presbyterian Church for the support you provided to the implementation phase of the Honoring Your Choices project.

The identified health care workers in the church community have agreed to be contacted and are available for any questions related to advanced care planning going forward.

This marks the end of the project. Thank you.

Sincerely,

Villeroy Tah, DNP Student

191 Springfield Street
Chicopee, MA 01013-2839
413-594-2761
www.elms.edu

Villeroy Tah, MSN, RN

Approval #121020211

January 30, 2022

Project Title: Honoring Your Choices

Site: HSPC Natick

Capstone Advisor: Dr. Teresa Kuta Reske

Dear ELMS College IRB Committee,

C/O Dr. Cynthia Dakin,

Thank you for working with me to ensure the implementation of this quality improvement project follows the ELMS IRB guidelines. The purpose of this letter is to notify you that the project was successfully implemented and was completed on December 12th, 2022, in accordance with the approved plan presented in the Proposal.

Sincerely,

Villeroy Tah

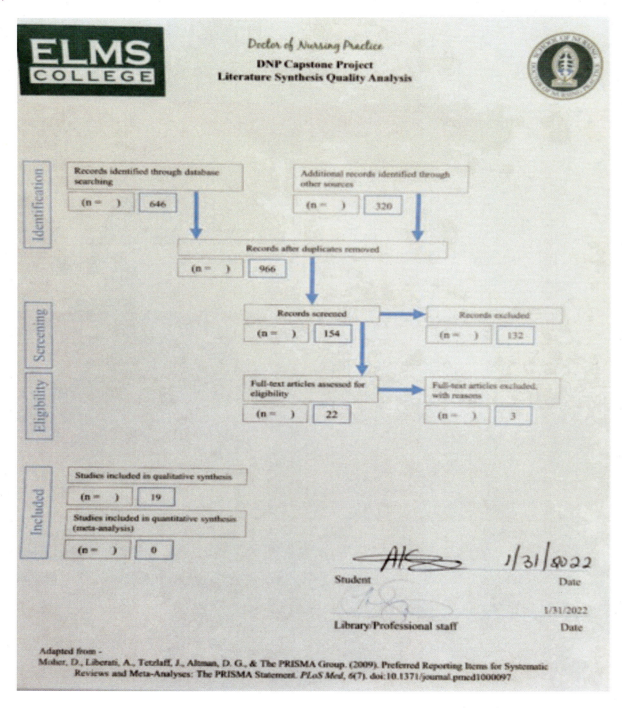

ELMS COLLEGE

Doctor of Nursing Practice
DNP Capstone Project
Literature Synthesis Quality Analysis

Identification

Records identified through database searching
(n =) 646

Additional records identified through other sources
(n =) 320

Records after duplicates removed
(n =) 966

Screening

Records screened
(n =) 154

Records excluded
(n =) 132

Eligibility

Full-text articles assessed for eligibility
(n =) 22

Full-text articles excluded, with reasons
(n =) 3

Included

Studies included in qualitative synthesis
(n =) 19

Studies included in quantitative synthesis (meta-analysis)
(n =) 0

Student _____ Date 1/31/2022

Library/Professional staff _____ Date 1/31/2022

Adapted from -
Moher, D., Liberati, A., Tetzlaff, J., Altman, D. G., & The PRISMA Group. (2009). Preferred Reporting Items for Systematic Reviews and Meta-Analyses: The PRISMA Statement. *PLoS Med, 6*(7). doi:10.1371/journal.pmed1000097

Table 1: Demographics for Participants

Demographics	Number (#) of Participants	# of Participants in Percentages
Ethnicity		
1. Black	26	83%
2. White	3	9.6%
3. Others	2	6.4%
Age		
1. 18 – 28	1	3.2%
2. 29 – 38	5	16.1%
3. 39 -48	7	22.6%
4. 49 – 58	10	32.2%
5. 59 – 68	4	13%
6. 69 – 78	3	9.7%
7. 79 – 88	0	0
8. 89 - above	0	0
Highest Level of Education		
1. High School or Less	7	22.6%
2. More than High School	23	74.2%
3. No Response	1	3.2%

	Survey Questions	Pre-Intervention (n = 30)			Post – Intervention (n = 31)		
	Questions	Agree	Disagree	No Response	Agree	Disagree	No Response
Q9.	I have the right to refuse medical treatment	**80.6%** (25)	19.4% (6)	0	**83.3%** (25)	17% (5)	0
Q10.	An HCP is someone who would make decisions on my behalf should…	**80.6%** (25)	16% (5)	3.2% (1)	**83.3%** (25)	10% (3)	6.7% (2)
Q11.	Once I sign an HCP, it cannot be changed	16% (5)	**74%** (23)	9.7% (3)	6.7% (2)	**86.7%** (26)	6.7% (2)
Q13.	An HCP is legal if only drawn up by a lawyer	6.5% (2)	**90%** (27)	6.5% (2)	6.7% (2)	86.7% (26)	6.7% (2)
Q14.	If I talked to my doctor, I don't need to talk to my family about my choices…	3.2% (1)	**93.5%** (29)	3.2% (1)	3.2% (1)	**90%** (27)	6.7% (2)

Table 3: Data Collection on Excel spreadsheets (details on pre- and post-survey results as broken down in the Appendices below)

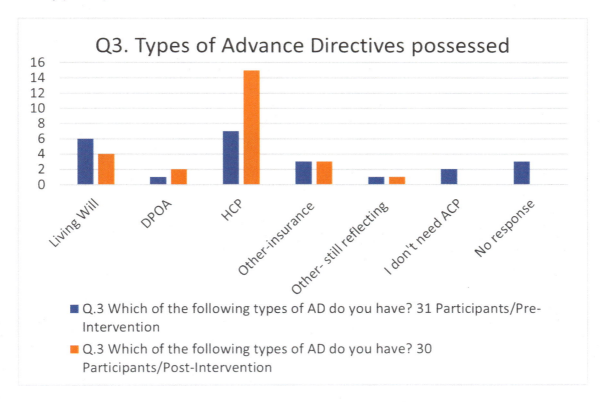

Figure 1: Pre and Post Intervention Survey Response to Q#3- Types of Advance Directives possessed by participants

Q3. Types of Advance Directives possessed

- Q.3 Which of the following types of AD do you have? 31 Participants/Pre-Intervention
- Q.3 Which of the following types of AD do you have? 30 Participants/Post-Intervention

Figure 2: Pre and Post Intervention Knowledge-based Q.s 9, 10 ,11 &13

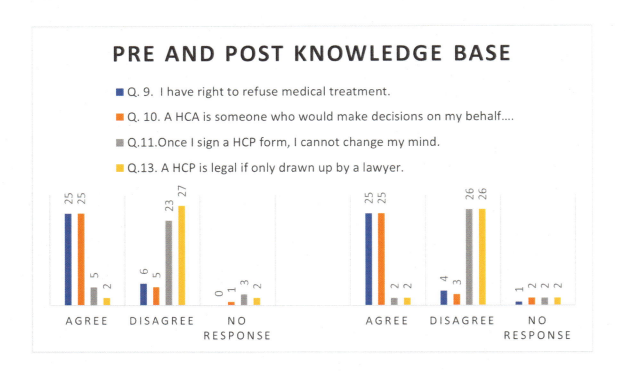

Figure 3: Post Intervention Response to Q 15- Status on HCP Completion

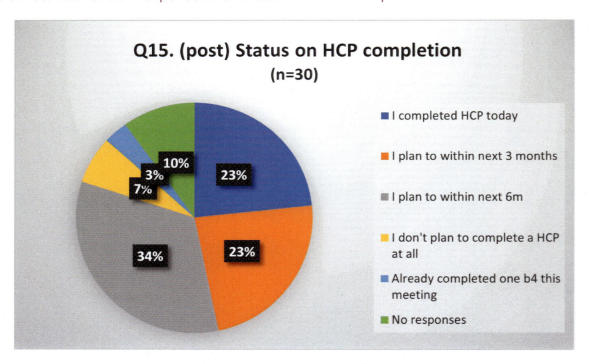

Figure 5: Pre and Post Intervention Survey Q1- Have you appointed an Health Care Proxy?

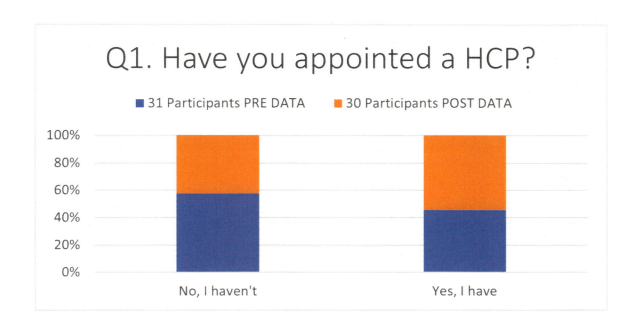

Figure 6: Pre and Post Intervention Survey Q2 – If you have already appointed a HCP, how long ago did you do this?

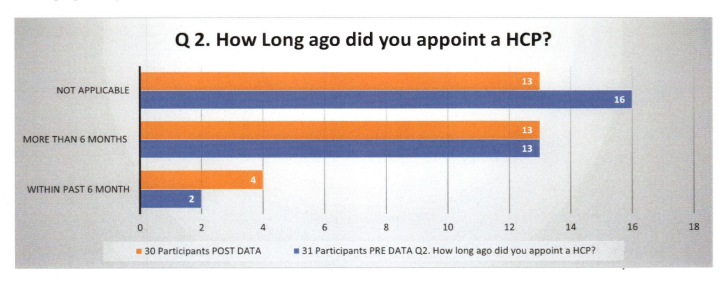

Figure 7: Pre and Post Intervention Survey Q4 – How long ago did you complete the HCP document?

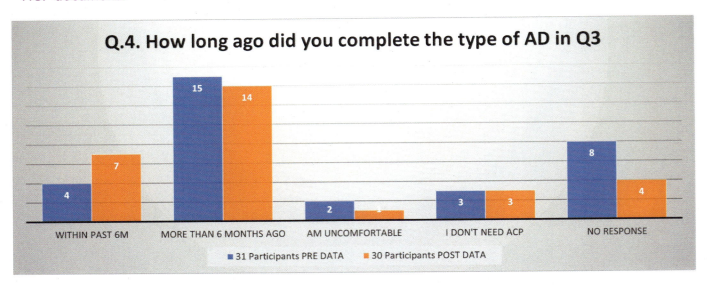

Figure 8: Pre and Post Intervention Survey Q5 – Have you talked to your family/friend about medical treatments that prolong life?

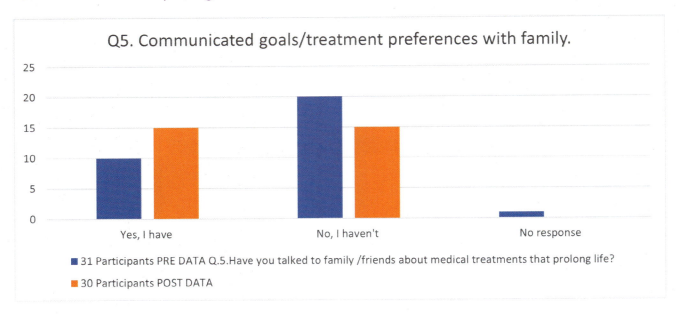

Figure 9: Pre and Post Intervention Survey Q6 – If you have already talked to your friend/ family about medical treatments that prolong life, how long ago did you do this?

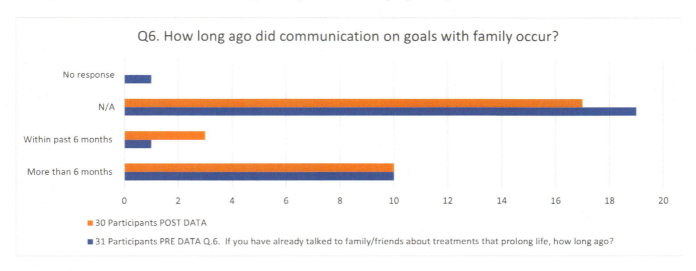

Q6. How long ago did communication on goals with family occur?

- 30 Participants POST DATA
- 31 Participants PRE DATA Q.6. If you have already talked to family/friends about treatments that prolong life, how long ago?

Figure 10: Pre and Post Intervention Survey Q7 – Have you talked to your doctor about what is important to you?

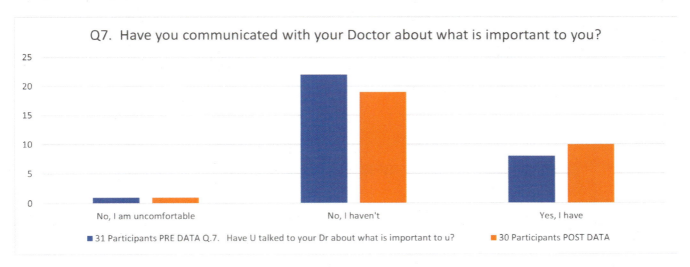

Q7. Have you communicated with your Doctor about what is important to you?

- 31 Participants PRE DATA Q.7. Have U talked to your Dr about what is important to u?
- 30 Participants POST DATA

Figure 11: If you already talked to your doctor about what is important to you, how long ago did you do this?

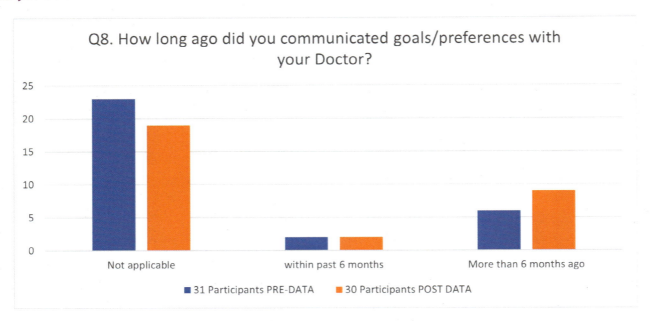

Figure 12: Pre and Post Intervention Knowledge-based Q 12 – Where is it important to keep a copy of an HCP?

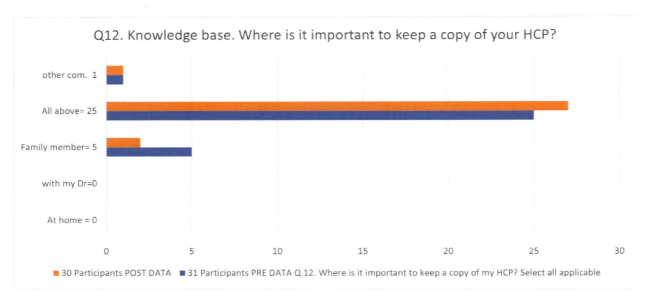

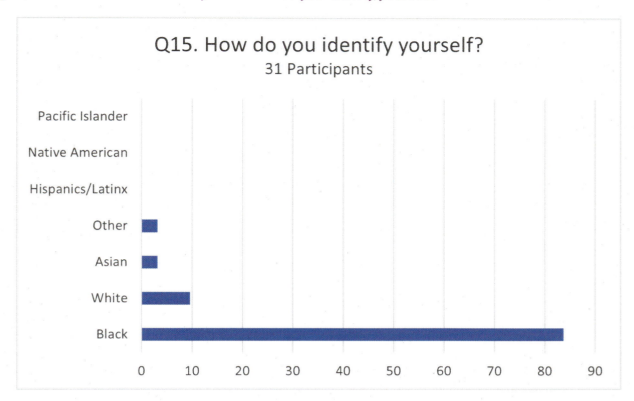

Figure 14: Pre-Intervention Survey Q16 - How old are you?

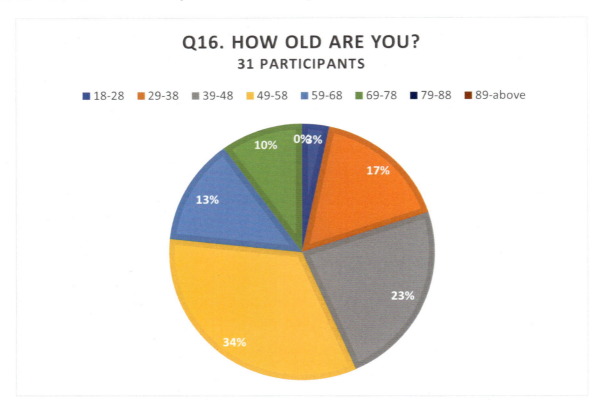

Q16. HOW OLD ARE YOU?
31 PARTICIPANTS

■ 18-28　■ 29-38　■ 39-48　■ 49-58　■ 59-68　■ 69-78　■ 79-88　■ 89-above

- 0%
- 3%
- 17%
- 23%
- 34%
- 13%
- 10%

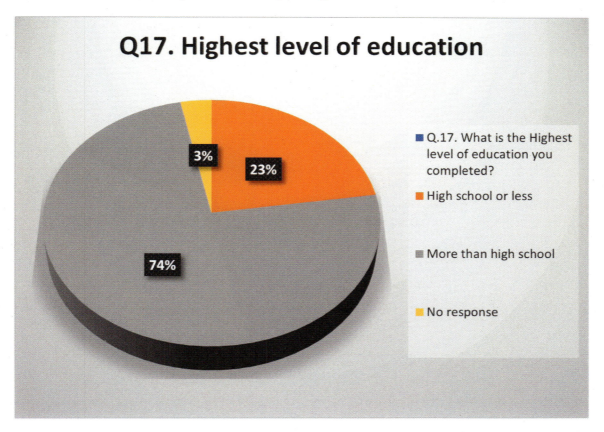

Conflict of interest: The author did not receive any grants for the implementation of the Honoring Your Choices quality improvement project or for this publication.